ANXIETY EXPLORATION 2-IN-1 BOX SET

ANXIETY MONSTER + HOARDING DISORDER HELP-
A GUIDE FOR MANAGING ANXIETY AND IT'S MANY
DISORDERS

MILTON HARRISON

CONTENTS

ANXIETY MONSTER

HOARDING DISORDER HELP

ANXIETY MONSTER

HOW TO MANAGE & LIVE WITH ANXIETY

INTRODUCTION

"You don't have to control your thoughts. You just have to stop letting them control you."

-   **Dan Millman**

"You don't have to control your thoughts. You just have to stop letting them control you."

— DAN MILLMAN

When walking down a lonely and dark alley and you notice a towering shadow tailing you, there will definitely be a reaction. Your defense mechanism will be at alert because you will start telling yourself, "What if this person is a robber or, worse, a killer?"

In such a scenario, the "fight or flight" hormone (adrenaline) will be released to help you think faster and act faster to evade the sensed danger. However, there is a side effect of this released adrenaline. It makes you anxious and scared, especially if you feel that person is going to hurt you.

The anxiety you develop in the scenario I just painted is totally normal. In fact, without anxiety, we will be unable to protect ourselves from danger. But as you know, everything has a limit. If your anxiety levels become more than normal, or persistent, or occur when there is little or no danger in sight, they become a problem. In such a case, your anxiety will bring about emotional distress and cause you great discomfort. That can disrupt your life by preventing you from doing the things you ought to do as a human being, such as associating with people, chasing a career, and living a life of freedom.

One can have a stress order and neglect it because they will conclude it is a natural phenomenon. They may feel that what they are experiencing is normal, and every other person gets to feel that way too. In this book, we will see the differences between normal worry and anxiety disorder for clarity's sake. This is important because if you don't identify these disorders for what they are and pursue treatment, they will be with you forever and go from bad to worse.

Anxiety can lead to depression, irrational fears, and even a physical panic, especially when you are in the midst of people. That is when we say that you have allowed your thoughts to control you. Dan Millman, in our opening quote, says it all. The truth is that thoughts will always be haphazard and spontaneous. You may find yourself going over one thought this minute, and the next minute, you will catch yourself grappling with an entirely new thought. That is because you and I cannot have absolute control over our thoughts. What we can do is allow the thoughts to do their things, but control the effect they have on us. If we can achieve that, we can say that we have prevented our thoughts from controlling us.

Over the years, I have gained a sound knowledge of anxiety and several other mental illnesses. I originally specialized in substance abuse, but my interest on how anxiety affects the human mind drove me into areas such as Obsessive-Compulsive Disorder (OCD), Social Anxiety Disorder (SAD), and General Anxiety Disorder (GAD), among several other subjects. In all of these, I have gathered tremendous knowledge and insight. In the course of this book, I will show you everything that my research and practice have taught me.

Why should you read this book? Do you know that anxiety disorders are the most prevalent mental illness in the U.S.? Statistics by Anxiety and Depression Association of America (ADAA) shows that every year, about 40 million adults aged 18 and above in the U.S. suffer from anxiety disorders. That's around 18.1% of the population. So even if you don't have it, there may be somebody you love who does. Even though this disease can be treated, people suffering from it hardly undergo treatment because they erroneously believe it is normal. Statistics say that only 36.9% of people suffering from the illness receive treatment.

The other 73.1% don't undergo treatment. On a worldwide scale, 75% of people who have depression and other mental illnesses in developing countries do not undergo treatment. The sad reality is that people do not realize that they can treat themselves from the comfort of their homes without spending a dime on any specialist. Yes, that is possible, and most of the people that I have taught and treated have been able to manage their anxiety effectively and live normal lives. There are several lifestyles, techniques, and strategies that you can adopt to cope with any anxiety you may have today.

In this book, we will look at the different types of anxiety disorders with an emphasis on the three most common ones —SAD, GAD, and OCD. We will look at the symptoms associated with them, the factors that trigger them, the coping strategies you can adopt, and so on. We will also discuss tested and trusted psychological remedies for them, such as Emotional Freedom Technique (EFT), mindfulness, and relaxation.

As you read this book, you should discover self-care methods that can help you manage that anxiety you thought was a life sentence. I will provide you with actionable steps that you can follow today to reclaim your freedom. I do not promise you an easy journey because it doesn't exist. At first, you will find it difficult to follow these steps, and it will seem as though it is not working at first, but with sheer determination, desire, and will, you will be amazed by how efficiently you can free yourself from the pangs of anxiety.

The quicker you act, the better for you. Anxiety disorders, just like most other mental illnesses, have a way of deteriorating if they are not treated quickly. Don't make the mistake of concluding that what you have is not an anxiety disorder. If you haven't been diagnosed with the disease, you have information in this book to use to conduct a self-check and know if you have any of these disorders or not. The key thing here is discovering early and acting accordingly before things spiral and depression sets it.

The remedies we will be discussing works because anxiety stems from our thoughts. If that is the case, then something can be done to reduce anxiety if we can work on our thoughts. When a troubling thought next hits your mind, and you catch yourself spiraling into anxiety and panic, know that you can stop those thoughts in their tracks. For instance, mindfulness and relaxation, some of the techniques we will be discussing, will teach you how to be in firm control of your mind by focusing on your present and drawing away from worries that you may have for the future or from a troubled past.

As you read through this book, my promise to you is that I am going to present everything in a language you will understand. I will not bore you with psychological jargon as that will only end up frightening you further. I hope that as you follow the tips and actionable steps I have provided in this book, you will regain your freedom in no time.

You never chose this path for yourself. You didn't just wake up one morning and wish for an anxiety disorder of any sort, but it is here nonetheless. That you have it now is not your fault, but if you choose not to do anything about it even when you can, that's when it becomes your fault.

I hope you make the right call today... See you on the anxiety-free side of life.

1

UNDERSTANDING ANXIETY AND ANXIETY DISORDERS

I n the introductory section of this book, we saw how it is okay for us to worry. When, then, should we be bothered, or to what magnitude should it occur before we make a move? In this chapter, we will take an in-depth look at anxiety, and we will also look at the various types of anxiety disorders out there.

My purpose in including this chapter is to help you know for sure if you have an anxiety disorder. For people who might have been diagnosed with the illness, this book will give you a better understanding of the illness you are suffering from. Whatever the case, I want you to realize that this is not a death sentence. It is totally manageable. Several people have done so, and you can do it too.

WHAT, THEN, IS ANXIETY?

Anxiety is a natural human emotion that is a crucial part of the fight or flight response. It can be likened to the alarm system in your house that alerts you when an intruder is on your property. The body's own alarm system is anxiety. It is what tells the body that an "intruder" is nearby. Anxiety and fear have been key to our survival as a species.

It occurs in response to those situations when we anticipate danger or something unpleasant happening. You don't expect the body not to defend itself, do you? Well, this is the first stage of the body defending itself. When anxiety sets in, the body weighs its option. In some cases, it decides to fight, but most times, it settles for flight, which simply means getting as far away as possible from the sensed danger. For instance, in the dark alley example we saw earlier, you have the option of seeing this one out (which is illogical, except maybe if you are a cop looking to catch a street robber), or speed up, or even run to where there are people and sufficient light. The physical responses we experience with anxiety are designed to help us respond to danger, preparing us to flee, fight, or freeze. It is known as the fight or flight response.

So anxiety, when occurring naturally in the right proportion, is not a problem because it is a natural human emotion, more or less like happiness, sadness, and every other human emotion that we express on a daily basis. This one is even a bit more important than other emotions, because thanks to anxiety, you have made it out of several dangerous situations in the past.

Anxiety does not only happen when we are in danger. It also occurs when we are under pressure or when we are faced with a difficult task. This is the reason why interviews, first dates, and public speaking are the greatest enemies that some people will ever know.

In light of this, it becomes obvious that anxiety does not just protect you from danger. Sometimes it serves different purposes, such as keeping you alert and focused, motivating you to solve problems, and spurring you to action.

The following are some of the signs associated with the fight or flight response:

Rapid heart rate & breathing

This is the body's way of preparing you for what is to come. For instance, if you ever fought that bully way back in high school, then you may recall how fast your heart was beating when you had been separated and asked the reason for your fight. My best bet is that you were unable to say a word, or you talked incoherently because you were still struggling to catch your breath.

The increased heart rate ensures that more energy and oxygen are supplied to the crucial body parts so that they can respond swiftly when the danger finally comes.

Pale or flushed skin

The skin becomes pale or flushed because the heart will starve the surface areas of the body blood so that it will supply the brains, muscles, arms, and legs with more blood. The reason is that these parts of the body will be busier when the body engages with the perceived danger. The blood clotting ability of the body also increases so that the body can prevent excessive loss of blood if the body gets injured as it engages with the perceived danger.

Dilated Pupils

Do you know that you see more when your body is in fight or flight mode? For instance, when you get into a fight, the eye becomes better at seeing so that it can watch for an incoming blow and warn you so you can respond suitably.

This is possible because when you are in danger, your pupils dilate to allow more light to get into the eyes. More light transcends to better vision and better response.

Trembling

Trembling occurs because when your body detects danger, it primes the muscles so that they can react quicker and better. It is this priming that causes shaking or trembling.

WHEN DOES IT BECOME A DISORDER?

When anxiety disrupts our lives and is present constantly, even when there is no genuine reason why it should be there, it has become an anxiety disorder and should be addressed in order to improve your quality of life.

Once anxiety begins to disrupt our life, we are in the territory of an anxiety disorder. That can mess with our stress hormones and fill the mind with toxic thoughts and worries. Such a situation will only push us into an even more anxious state.

As you would expect, there are levels of anxiety disorder. Some sufferers may have chronic anxiety disorders that throw them into fits of panic, so they literally shake when they are anxious. Others might experience a mild case, such as doing everything possible to avoid crowded places or trembling at the mic when it is time to speak before a group of people.

Anxiety disorder is a general label to cover various debilitating conditions. There are seven main ones, three of which will be explored more closely in the book. Some of the disorders are not a single disorder but a group of related conditions.

WHAT CAUSES ANXIETY DISORDERS?

Researchers have not been able to pinpoint a particular thing as the cause of anxiety disorders. For now, the general consensus is that a combination of factors contributes to the disorder. The common factors that have been identified for now are genetics and environmental factors, as well as an individual's brain chemistry.

KEY THINGS YOU SHOULD KNOW ABOUT ANXIETY DISORDER

Recent surveys suggest we live in an "age of anxiety" in which modern life plays a pivotal role and could be responsible for the rise in anxiety disorders.

Research into the parts of the brain involved with anxiety is ongoing.

There is no single test to diagnose an anxiety disorder. Diagnosis involves a long process involving physical examinations, mental health evaluations, and psychological questionnaires.

Anxiety disorders often co-occur with depression, but not always.

Anxiety disorders are a group of interrelated conditions (not a single disorder), and symptoms vary.

Anxiety disorders are some of the most common forms of mental health issues and can be managed with the right information and tools.

WHAT ARE THE LIKELY SYMPTOMS?

You may have an anxiety disorder if:

- You are constantly worried or tense.
- Your anxiety interferes with your work, education, or relationships.
- You can't shake off what you know to be irrational fears.
- You think something bad will happen if things aren't done in a particular way.
- You avoid situations because they cause you anxiety.
- You experience sudden attacks of panic.
- You feel like danger is around every corner.

These symptoms manifest them in two ways: psychological and physical.

The symptoms that are mostly psychological/emotional are:

- Feelings of dread
- Watching for signs of danger
- Expecting the worst
- Difficulty concentrating
- Feeling tense
- Irritability
- Blank mind, especially when before people

The physical ones that are caused by the body being flooded by the stress hormone known as cortisol include:

- Pounding heart
- Sweats
- Headaches
- Stomach ache
- Dizziness
- Shaking or trembling
- Frequent urination or diarrhea.
- Frequent bathroom trips
- Shortness of breath
- Tension in muscles
- Insomnia

Because of the similarity of these symptoms with those of other diseases, sufferers of anxiety disorder usually mistake their illness for other medical illnesses depending on the symptoms that are prevalent. For instance, if a person comes down with a stomach ache and gets diarrhea too, you will need to go the extra mile as a therapist to convince them that it is not diarrhea but an anxiety disorder. This has caused several people with anxiety disorders to truly never notice.

ANXIETY SYMPTOMS AND DEPRESSION

These two are almost becoming synonymous because they are often seen together. If you are suffering from anxiety symptoms, it won't be long before depression sets in. For instance, if you are suffering from a chronic social anxiety disorder, my best bet is that you prefer to lock yourself in your apartment all day long. A condition like that precedes depression because sooner or later, you will start telling yourself that you are not good enough to associate with people. You will convince yourself that you are incomplete, unlike other people. At that stage, depression sets in, and that is when some people cannot handle it anymore, and take their lives.

The presence of depression worsens anxiety symptoms and vice versa.

TYPES OF ANXIETY DISORDER

There are seven types of anxiety disorder. In the course of this book, we will discuss the three most common types of anxiety disorder: SAD, GAD, and OCD. I have dedicated three chapters to them so that we won't be discussing them extensively in this chapter. Discussions on GAD, SAD, and OCD can be found in chapters four, five, and six, respectively. So in this chapter, we will give more attention to those disorders that we may never mention again.

But first, let's remind ourselves of what the three main disorders are:

Generalized Anxiety Disorder (GAD)

This type of anxiety is characterized by worries and fear. It makes you have that persistent feeling that something terrible will happen. If you have noticed that you are a chronic worrywart who always gets this anxious feeling over most things at most times, then you may be suffering from GAD. If you are truly honest with yourself, you will agree with me that most times you don't even know why you are worried. Even when there is a reason, it is hardly substantial enough to elicit such a reaction from you.

This disorder is mostly characterized by symptoms such as restlessness, fatigue, insomnia, and stomach upset.

We will discuss GAD in more detail in chapter four of this book.

Social Anxiety Disorder (SAD)

This order is mostly the fear of socializing with people because you are scared that their view of you might be negative, and you might be humiliated in public. Another name for this disorder is social phobia, which translates to fear of social settings. It is extreme shyness that keeps its sufferers from living their lives to the fullest.

Sufferers prefer to keep to themselves always and associate only when it is inevitable. In extreme cases, the sufferer will withdraw totally from all forms of social gathering. The problem with that is that you need to interact with people to make any headway in life. You need to go to school, be a part of a class, and undertake projects in school before you can graduate. And when you do, you need to take up a job and communicate with your coworkers. Even if you are starting your digital business from your home, at some point you will need to make presentations. You need to relieve yourself of some stress by spending quality time with family or friends. But with SAD, all of these things will elude you.

SAD will be discussed in more detail in chapter five.

. . .

Obsessive-Compulsive Disorder (OCD)

This disorder is characterized by recurring irrational thoughts that can cause the sufferer to perform specific behaviors in a repetitive manner. It also causes undesired behaviors and thoughts that you cannot control. In extreme cases, a sufferer may experience uncontrollable compulsions like washing their face time and time again without any need for such actions. In some people, it is a recurring worry that they have left something undone that needed to be done. For instance, a sufferer may erroneously believe that they left their door open on their way out of the house earlier that day when, in fact, they locked up everywhere accordingly.

OCD will be discussed in more detail in chapter six.

Panic Disorder

Panic disorder, also known as a panic attack, is characterized by sudden, repeated panic attacks and the fear of experiencing the attack again. This fear of experiencing the attack again can be more debilitating than the actual attack itself. Panic disorder is often associated with agoraphobia, which is the fear of being in a place where it might be difficult to escape or get help in a difficult event. People with agoraphobia will avoid confined spaces such as airplanes.

PHOBIAS AND IRRATIONAL FEARS

These are characterized by an exaggerated and intense fear of specific things, places, or situations. This fear is termed irrational because, oftentimes, the actual danger is way less than what the sufferer senses it to be.

Some of the most common phobias are fear of animals, heights, enclosed space, or flying. Sufferers of these phobias will do everything possible to avoid those things they are scared of. The result is a continual and increasing fear of that thing. Before the sufferer can overcome their fears, they must face their fears and see for themselves that they had been exaggerating.

My guess is that you never thought phobias were mental illnesses. Well, now you know. So if you have one of those misplaced fears, it is time to rid yourself of it.

Post-Traumatic Stress Disorder (PTSD)

This is an extreme anxiety disorder that is the result of traumatic events in the life of the sufferer. It can also be caused by life-threatening situations in which the sufferer never thought they would survive. When the traumatic or life-threatening situation is gone, the sufferer is not able to erase it from their mind. So it remains there and torments them until they do something about it.

It is a condition that is very common with war veterans because they had seen horrible things when they were fighting in wars. They are never able to erase these terrible memories, and it manifests itself as PTSD.

The common systems are nightmares, hypervigilance, quick startling, flashbacks, and a strong desire to avoid situations that can remind the sufferer of the memories that haunts them.

Separation Anxiety Disorder

This disorder is most common in children. It is normal for children not to want to be separated from their parents, but if the anxiety associated with the separation intensifies, it becomes a problem. If you notice that your child becomes agitated at the thought of being separated from you, they may have a separation anxiety disorder.

In summary, anxiety, when occurring moderately and naturally, is good. And you must learn to pay close attention whenever you catch yourself feeling anxious. But if it becomes too much that it now interferes with your activities and wellbeing, you must seek a solution. There are no carved-in-stone symptoms for any of the anxiety disorders. So your symptoms might be different from those of your neighbor with the same condition. That is because anxiety disorders are mostly a combination of several disorders, not just one.

Later in this book, I will show you several self-care routines that you can adopt in your fight against anxiety disorders. It is totally curable. The key thing is getting to know what your disorders are. And do not go hard on yourself for having any anxiety disorders. Realize that you are not alone; so many others have it and are living life as they should, so do not limit yourself from achieving what you are able.

2

A CLOSER LOOK AT ANXIETY ATTACKS

W e often confuse panic attacks with anxiety attacks, but there are differences between them. The two main reasons they are mistaken for each other is that anxiety attacks aren't medically recognized, and panic attacks are often experienced by those living with anxiety.

I will explain how they are related, so you have a better understanding.

ANXIETY ATTACK AND PANIC ATTACK, HOW DO THEY RELATE?

In my years of practice, I've seen people use anxiety attacks and panic attacks interchangeably. They just assume they are alternate names for a single disorder. But that is not the case because even though they have their similarities, they have significant differences.

The main reason why people tend to mistake them for each other is that they share some common symptoms, and these symptoms can be experienced simultaneously or concurrently. For instance, worrying about a stressful meeting can cause anxiety, which may culminate as a panic attack during the meeting. In this case, we see how it is possible for one attack to stem from another one.

People who experience anxiety attacks are more likely to have panic attacks. But that doesn't mean that everybody with an anxiety disorder will get a panic disorder. It is possible to live with an anxiety disorder and never experience a panic attack.

It may be that if you live with an anxiety disorder, panic attacks are part of your experience. They usually peak within ten minutes and last less than 30 minutes. They can be very frightening, sometimes with symptoms so severe that they feel like a heart attack.

PANIC ATTACKS

Panic attacks can be destabilizing for its sufferer. When it occurs, you will be scared because you will feel like you are losing control or going crazy. In extreme cases, you may even conclude that you have a heart attack that may kill you. But on its own, a panic attack is not life-threatening.

If you experience a panic attack once or twice in a lifetime, it doesn't mean that you have panic disorder. Many people will experience the occasional panic attack, but this doesn't mean they have panic disorder. It only becomes a panic disorder when the panic attack is recurrent, and you notice that you are living in fear that you might experience another attack shortly. It is this fear that is even more damaging because you will do all you can to avoid situations that you feel may lead to another attack. This has caused several people living with panic disorder to avoid work, school, and other social gatherings. With such a routine, it becomes very difficult for the individual to reach their true potential in life.

A panic attack can occur anywhere or at any time without warning. It can happen when you are fast asleep, at work, driving, or at the mall. It is believed that when a particular event causes you to have a panic attack, that event has a way of making you feel endangered and trapped. When your mind has set itself on this belief even when it might not be true, it causes your body to go into the fight or flight mode. (We discussed the fight and flight mode earlier.) As your body enters that mode, it manifests most of the responses that your body would normally manifest when it is in actual danger.

There are several variations in symptoms. This means that the symptoms you will get, and their duration will differ from that of someone else. Irrespective of the variations, the attack and resultant symptoms usually peak within minutes. After you recover from the panic attack, you may feel exhausted, as though you just did a tedious task.

The intense fear you feel during the attack can mar your self-confidence and disrupt your everyday life, depending on the intensity of the attack. It can cause the following panic disorder symptoms:

- Anticipatory Anxiety: This is the constant fear you have in-between episodes that prevent you from being your normal self, even when the panic is not upon you. It affects your efficiency at every other thing because it can be disabling.
- Phobic Avoidance: This is the name for the avoidance I talked about. You may believe that the situation you are avoiding was the cause of your previous attack. Hence, you will do everything you can to never be in that condition again.

HOW TO OVERCOME FEAR OF PANIC ATTACK

In your attempt to reduce panic attack episodes, you will need to have a strong answer to anticipatory anxiety that we discussed above. Again, it is the way you respond to the unpleasant situation that determines the extent to which the panic attack will affect you.

Most people react to the unpleasant situation by convincing themselves that they cannot control themselves, or that they are having a heart attack. Some people will even conclude that they are going insane or, in the worst-case scenario, that they are dying. All of these conclusions will just escalate the fear in them and cause symptoms to increase until they get out of hand.

You can overcome your fear by:

1. Educating yourself

By reading this book, you are already doing some of what is necessary. It is better when you recognize panic disorder for what it is because that will eliminate some of the misplaced fear such as, "I am going to die," or "I am going insane" that people usually have when they have panic attacks. You should eliminate these fears because they always escalate your symptoms.

As you educate yourself and recognize the likely symptoms, you will identify them for what they truly are.

2. Don't live in denial

After educating yourself, accept your panic attacks. Don't try to resist the symptoms as that can worsen your situation by increasing your fear and anxiety. The idea here is that when you accept your panic attacks, you will alter your perception of the attacks. That is when you can cope because you begin to see it as a natural phenomenon, and not a curse that has come to ruin you.

3. Change your response

When you have accepted your panic attacks, the next thing you should change is the response you give to panic attacks. Instead of responding with fear, anxiety, and negative beliefs, start to respond with calmness, clarity, and control.

These three responses can be regarded as the Three A's: Acknowledge, Accept, and give Alternative responses. In the acknowledgment stage of this process, you are expected to be calm and recognize the experience. In the acceptance, try to come to terms with the fact that you are in the middle of a panic attack. Finally, in the alternative response, tell yourself that the feelings you are experiencing are just temporary.

SOME CHARACTERISTICS OF PANIC ATTACK

- It comes on suddenly and involves intense/overwhelming fear.
- It comes with physical symptoms such as a racing heart, shortness of breath, or nausea.
- It is recognized by the Diagnostic and Statistical Manual of Mental Disorders (DSM-5).
- It may not always be cued by stressors—it may come out of the blue. But expected panic attacks are cued by external stressors, such as phobias.
- Severe, disruptive symptoms—fight or flight response—takes over.
- It often triggers fears related to having another attack.

SOME CHARACTERISTICS OF ANXIETY ATTACKS:

- Aren't recognized by the DSM-5
- May come on gradually.
- Lack of diagnostic recognition makes them harder to define by symptoms.

- It is typically related to something perceived as stressful.
- It can be mild, moderate, or severe, and builds gradually.

DIFFERENCES BETWEEN ANXIETY ATTACK AND PANIC ATTACK

The differences between the symptoms of an anxiety attack and panic attack can be classified into emotional and physical.

Emotional:

An anxiety attack is characterized by apprehension and worry, distress, restlessness, and fear, while a panic attack is characterized by fear. This may include fear of dying or losing control, or a sense of detachment from the world.

Physical:

In terms of physical symptoms, there is hardly a clear difference between them. The only difference is in the severity, with a panic attack generally being more severe. The physical symptoms are explained in the next section.

SYMPTOMS OF PANIC ATTACK

A panic disorder showcases itself in the form of a panic attack. The symptoms associated with a panic attack can cut across the physical, emotional, and cognitive aspects of a patient.

If you have experienced the following, you may have had a panic attack:

Heart palpitations.

Heart palpitation is one of the greatest sources of fear for people experiencing panic attacks. They will erroneously believe that the accelerated heart rate they are experiencing is caused by either a heart attack or other medical emergencies.

But that is not the case. An accelerated heart rate can occur due to several reasons, such as excitement and natural nervousness. When your heart beats fast due to excitement, you are calm and collected, but when it happens during a panic attack, you interpret it as a heart attack, and that is the problem.

As we will see later in this book, simple exercises, such as deep breathing, can put you back in control.

Shaking.

During a panic attack, you may experience trembling sensations, which will show as shaky legs, arms, hands, and feet. This can really frighten you, but on closer inspection, you will realize that these are normal body reactions to fight or flight mode.

Excessive Sweating.

The sweating you experience is caused by the anxious feeling that you are having. It is the way our body responds to stress. If you didn't know this, you could interpret it to mean a very serious emergency.

This sweating may be accompanied by chills or hot flashes. It may be hot sweat or cold sweat. Whichever way it comes, realize that it is just the body's way of responding to stress.

Hyperventilation.

During a panic attack, you may not be able to breathe the way you do when you are calm. You may notice that instead of having calm, rhythmic breathing, you take quick, short breaths. It can be really frightening because you can feel like you're about to choke.

Apart from these major symptoms, other common ones are:

- Feeling faint
- Trouble breathing
- Hot flashes or chills
- Overwhelming panic
- Loss of control
- Nausea
- Feeling detached

Risk factors include:

- Experiencing or witnessing trauma in the past
- Experiencing a stressful life event
- Ongoing stress and worry
- Living with a chronic health condition
- Having another mental health disorder
- Substance use
- Anxiety or panic disorders in the family

TYPES OF PANIC ATTACK

Not everybody who suffers a panic attack experiences the same type of attack. The symptoms associated with the different types of attacks may be similar, but the causes will differ.

The three recognized type of panic attacks are:

1. Unexpected (Un-cued) Panic Attacks

These types of attacks come upon the sufferer without any signal, warning, or trigger. It is a rapid attack that seems to come out of thin air. If you suffer from an unexpected panic attack, you may go into a full state of panic without any clear cause. You may not be doing anything that could lead to an attack, yet, it will still arise. Due to its nature, this type of attack cannot be predicted; neither can you prepare for it. Since this attack occurs without any situational or environmental trigger, it can even happen while you are asleep.

At the time of the attack, patients will normally experience symptoms such as a rapid heartbeat or rise in body temperature and may feel the need to leave where they are at the time of the attack.

2. Situational Bound or Cued Panic Attacks:

This type of attack occurs when you are exposed to certain situations. Once you have suffered a panic attack over a situation, that situation is likely to become a cue or trigger for subsequent panic episodes. For instance, if you have a fear of social gatherings, and it has led you to a panic attack before, you may suffer another episode when you are in a social gathering. You may also suffer an attack just by thinking about a social gathering. For you, work meetings, family gatherings, interviews, religious gatherings, and parties become a no-no because you know it can trigger another episode.

Due to their nature, they are more predictable. But this predictability itself is a demerit to you because when you are aware that you might suffer a panic attack, the chances of it happening will increase. That is because the fear and anxiety you have that it may happen can be extremely overwhelming, and you can only hold in there for so long before you give in to the tension.

3. Situationally Predisposed Panic Attacks:

This type of attack is actually caused by triggers, but the attack does not occur immediately upon exposure. It will lead to delayed attack, happening after you have been exposed to the trigger several times. This means that a person with a social anxiety disorder may not experience a panic disorder at a social gathering, but upon continuous exposure or after leaving the social gathering, they may suffer an attack.

For instance, if somebody's trigger for an attack is flying, they may not experience an attack while they are flying, but when they get off the plane or even get home, they may have a panic attack.

This type of attack is a bit more complex than the others because a panic attack might or might not occur on exposure to triggers.

CAUSES OF PANIC ATTACK

As at the time of writing this book, the medical world has not been able to clearly identify the exact cause of panic attacks and panic disorders. However, it is believed that it can be hereditary.

The items listed below are the possible causes of expected panic attacks since the unexpected ones don't have external triggers. Also, note that these causes can also trigger an anxiety attack. The triggers are:

- Stressful tasks, such as tough jobs.
- Driving.
- Social situations.
- Phobias such as claustrophobia or agoraphobia.
- Memories of past traumatic experiences.
- Chronic illnesses, such as heart diseases, diabetes, and asthma.
- Chronic pain.
- Caffeine (I will show you how this can trigger a panic attack in chapter three when we start discussing lifestyle changes you should try).

- Medication and supplements.
- Thyroid problems.

Apart from the causes above, panic attacks can also be caused by medical conditions.

DIAGNOSIS

Doctors cannot diagnose anxiety attacks, but panic attacks, alongside anxiety symptoms, anxiety disorders, and panic disorders can be diagnosed. Before diagnosis, the doctor will ask you what symptoms you've noticed. If these are in line with some of the symptoms we've identified above, the doctor will conduct other tests to rule out the possibility that your symptoms are due to illnesses other than a panic attack. For instance, heart diseases and thyroid problems have some symptoms that are similar to panic attack symptoms.

To be sure it is really a panic disorder, you may have to see a doctor who will conduct relevant tests to rule out the following possibilities:

1. Mitral valve prolapses. This is a minor cardiac problem that is a result of the inefficiency of one of the heart valves.
2. Hyperthyroidism. This is a medical condition that is caused by an overactive thyroid gland.

3. Hyperglycemia. This is a condition caused by low blood sugar.

The usual tests that you would expect a doctor to perform are a physical examination, blood tests, a psychological evaluation, and heart tests such as an electrocardiogram (ECG or EKG).

Whatever the result of your analysis, don't panic over it. Know that there are several home remedies that can reduce or stop the symptoms altogether. We will discuss them in subsequent chapters. Keep reading to discover them.

DEALING WITH AN ANXIETY OR PANIC ATTACK

- Take slow, deep breaths, focusing your attention on every breath. Count to four as you exhale, and repeat until breathing slows.
- Recognize and accept the attack. Remind yourself that it will pass.
- Practice mindfulness. This will be discussed in detail in chapter eight of this book.
- Use relaxation techniques. In chapter nine of this book, we will discuss this in detail.

We will discuss these coping strategies later in this book.

Prevention

It may not be feasible to prevent attacks completely, but you can reduce the severity and frequency by:

- Reducing or taking out the sources of stress in your life.
- Learning to identify and stop negative thoughts.
- Practice meditation.
- Join a support group.
- Make lifestyle changes. Lifestyle changes such as exercising, eating healthy, and sleeping correctly, are some lifestyle changes that can help improve your condition. (We will talk more on this in chapter 3.)

Medication

While a panic attack itself cannot be treated with medication, some of the associated symptoms can. So a doctor might recommend medication for these treatable symptoms.

The common medications for panic disorder symptoms are:

Antidepressants: This medication works best when a person living with panic disorder is also experiencing symptoms of depression. The common antidepressants are serotonin reuptake inhibitors (SSRI) such as Prozac (fluoxetine) and Zoloft (sertraline).

Anti-anxiety medications: This medication may ease anxiety by acting as a depressant on the central nervous system. Common examples are benzodiazepines, such as Xanax.

LONG-TERM OUTLOOK

Unfortunately, panic disorder is a long-term condition, and it may be challenging to treat. While some people with this illness may react to medical treatments, most won't. Those who respond may enter a period of no symptoms, but they can spiral into periods of intense symptoms. However, changes in diet, sleeping patterns, and relaxation techniques can help. I will show you how.

Summarily, anxiety attacks and panic attacks are not the same as most people think. One of the significant differences is that while a panic attack is identified in DSM-5 as a mental disorder, an anxiety attack is not. While the two ailments share similar symptoms, triggers, and risk factors, panic attacks tend to be more intense and can bring severe physical symptoms with it, unlike anxiety attacks.

Whatever your condition may be, I want you to find solace in the fact that they both can be treated. Irrespective of what the cause may be and the way it manifests itself, you can gradually eliminate the symptoms of the panic so you can regain your confidence and live your best life.

In the next chapter, we will be going deeper as I will be introducing the value of a healthy lifestyle.

3

BUILDING ON STRONG FOUNDATIONS: THE VALUE OF A HEALTHY LIFESTYLE

I n the fight against every form of anxiety, having a strong foundation is an excellent place to start. Having a strong foundation means you are living a healthy lifestyle. In this chapter, I will show you all the great ways you can reduce anxiety by living a healthy life. I will not just show you what you have to do; I will also show you the benefits you can get from doing them.

Lifestyle changes may not completely cure an anxiety disorder. Still, if you live with anxiety, you can make changes to your diet, your exercise routine, sleep, and social patterns that can help reduce symptoms and help you manage your anxiety on the day-to-day. Ensuring your lifestyle is healthy and balanced across all of these elements can give you a strong foundation on which to build other factors to reduce anxiety.

Whether you have an anxiety disorder or you live with milder or less persistent anxiety, lifestyle changes can help improve your symptoms. If you lead an unhealthy lifestyle, you are more likely to experience anxiety.

Now let's see some of your life areas that you can tweak today to help you overcome anxiety disorder no matter the form it takes.

DIET

There are indications that some foods can help reduce the symptoms of anxiety, and some can increase anxiety and intensify physical symptoms.

For instance, alcohol and caffeine are notoriously bad for anxiety patients, likewise fatty foods. When you reduce your fatty foods intake and take enough calcium, zinc, a lot of fresh foods such as vegetables, and plenty of water, it will help reduce the symptoms. Many other dietary options can help in relieving anxiety, and we will discuss them extensively in this chapter.

At the basic level, a balanced diet and staying hydrated can help relieve anxiety, but specific diets can do even more for you in your fight against anxiety. They include:

. . .

1. Complex carbohydrates

Complex carbohydrates are metabolized slowly during diges-tion, and that can help you stabilize your blood sugar level, which creates a calmer feeling. Complex carbohydrates include fruits, whole grains, and vegetables. A diet rich in whole grain, vegetables, and fruits is healthier and recom-mended rather than eating simple carbohydrates found in processed foods. That means fast foods and junks may not be the right call at this point in your life because they lack complex carbohydrates. Stick to the ones mentioned here or have a nutritionist plan your meal to afford you more complex carbohydrates daily.

2. Foods that Prompt The Release of Neurotrans-mitters:

Certain foods are even more important for people with anxiety disorders. For instance, the following foods prompt the release of neurotransmitters (e.g., serotonin and dopamine), which can improve anxiety symptoms.

Probiotics

Probiotics are important because they improve gut health. That is because the gut-brain axis, the lining precisely, contains 95% of serotonin receptors. Examples of probiotics are pickles, kefir, and yogurt.

Foods with a high magnesium content

Magnesium is a crucial mineral in the body. It plays an important role in many bodily functions, along with other health benefits. It is very helpful as a natural treatment for anxiety. In an experiment designed to learn more about the relationship between magnesium and anxiety, diets low in magnesium caused test mice to exhibit more anxiety-related behaviors. It was concluded that foods rich in magnesium could induce feelings of calmness in both mice and humans. One of the reasons why magnesium might reduce anxiety is that it can improve brain function. It does that by regulating neurotransmitters, which send messages throughout the body. Magnesium also improves brain functions that reduce stress and anxiety. It is a part of the brain called the hypothalamus. The hypothalamus regulates the pituitary and adrenal glands, which controls the body's response to stress. These are all reasons why you need to have enough magnesium in your diet. Examples of foods rich in magnesium are leafy greens, legumes, nuts and seeds, and whole grains.

Foods high in zinc:

Zinc is an important mineral that aids in cell development and expression of genes. Many people misunderstand the importance of zinc in mental health disorders. The body needs zinc to make neurotransmitters, and without zinc, a neurotransmitter imbalance can cause symptoms of anxiety. It is important we take a proper balance of neurotransmitters such as GABA, norepinephrine, dopamine, and serotonin. The neurotransmitter that affects mood, appetite, sleep, digestion, libido, and memory is primarily serotonin. Norepinephrine is a stress hormone. It is released from the sympathetic nervous system in response to stress. GABA is connected to anxiety. Dopamine is mostly found in the brain and affects your emotions, sensations of pleasure and pain, and movement. So it is necessary to take foods high in zinc such as cashews, liver, oysters, beef, and egg yolks. Foods having omega-3 fatty acids such as salmon and mackerel also have good zinc content and can help reduce anxiety symptoms.

Foods high in B vitamins

Foods containing B vitamins are essential when trying to reduce anxiety levels. That is because Vitamin B helps balance blood sugar levels, which is a significant factor in controlling anxiety. Vitamin B is grouped into eight separate vitamins, and each is essential. Vitamin B5 helps the adrenal glands that reduce anxiety levels and stress. Vitamin B12 and vitamin B9 are needed for reducing depression. Vitamin B6 and magnesium can both help reduce anxiety. Vitamin B3 helps in the synthesis of serotonin and has been shown to help with anxiety. Foods high in vitamin B include avocados, bananas, potatoes, liver, nutritional yeast, and almonds.

Asparagus

Asparagus has anti-anxiety properties. Asparagus is rich in fiber, potassium, and vitamins A, C, E, and K, and its beneficial trace is well-known to reduce anxiety. It is also known as a mood enhancer. It is so effective against anxiety that the Chinese government approved it for use in beverages.

3. Foods High in Antioxidants

Research shows that anxiety is caused when a body has a lowered antioxidant state, increasing foods high in antioxidants can help. A 2010 study showed the antioxidant content of 3,100 supplements, beverages, spices, herbs, and foods. That study was conducted because it is common knowledge that antioxidants can reduce the risk of oxidative stress-related diseases.

The United States Department of Agriculture (USDA) stipulates that the foods listed below are high in antioxidant content:

- Beans such as red kidney, black, pinto, and small dried red.
- Fruits such as apples, prunes, sweet cherries, and black plums.

- Berries such as strawberries, blackberries, cranberries, raspberries, and blueberries.
- Nuts such as walnuts and pecans.
- Vegetables such as spinach, beet, broccoli, and kale.

Foods alone will not eliminate your anxiety disorder, but there is growing evidence that shows a strong connection between nutrition and psychiatry. Studies are still ongoing, but from what we see already, the future linking healthy foods and healthy minds is positive.

Meal timing

The diets recommended above can be more effective for you if you don't skip meals. When you skip meals, your blood sugar may drop, and this can cause you to feel jittery, worsening any underlying anxiety. It can have other consequences, which also increase anxiety. For instance, complex carbohydrates stabilize your blood sugar but ask yourself what will happen if you have a meal rich in carbohydrates, but you skipped breakfast and lunch.

In essence, the meals mentioned are most efficient when you are consistent with them.

THINGS TO AVOID

Just as some food items can help relieve your symptoms, there are some that you should try to minimize because they can worsen your condition. Cutting certain foods out altogether can also be beneficial.

Let's look at some of the things you should reduce or cut out entirely from your diet so that you can further reduce your anxiety episodes and the severity of the symptoms you will suffer in the once-in-a-while episodes.

Caffeine

If you are a lover of coffee, I know this point will not appeal to you. Some people have told me how they will want to try every other thing I have recommended, but not this one. But the truth is, you have no other choice but to cut down or totally forgo those coffee breaks. Excessive consumption of caffeine can trigger anxiety and aggravate symptoms; it does this by increasing the activity around the sympathetic nervous system. Also, caffeine is known to be a stimulant and can worsen an anxious patient's condition by triggering an anxiety attack. When someone with anxiety takes caffeine, it blocks the adenosine that makes you feel tired and triggers the release of adrenaline that increases energy, thereby keeping you in the "fight or flight" mode we talked about earlier.

Do you know that if you consume over 200 mg of caffeine, this can increase your likelihood of having a panic or anxiety attack? Excessive consumption of caffeine has also been shown to result in symptoms ranging from symptoms of General Anxiety Disorder (GAD) to phobic, and obsessive-compulsive symptoms.

Coffee is not the only food that has high caffeine content. Other foods and drinks that may have high caffeine content are sodas, candies, coffee liqueurs, green tea, dark chocolate, and energy drinks.

Withdrawal symptoms of caffeine: If caffeine is a big part of your diet, stopping it at once could have a bad effect on you in the short-term. The effects that you might encounter include sleepiness, tiredness, headache, down moods, difficulty in concentration, and so on. These symptoms might start within two or three days from when you stopped taking it. So you should stop it gradually by reducing the quantity bit by bit until you are used to not taking it.

But if you must take it, keep it as minimal as possible. To avoid the negative effects of caffeine on your health, you should consume one 12-ounce coffee or one shot of espresso (about 350mg a day) daily, nothing more than that.

Timing matters too. Taking coffee in the dead of night is all shades of wrong. Some people ignorantly harm themselves by drinking caffeine at 12:00 pm. Taking caffeine by this time or beyond can cause severe harm to your health and increase your anxiety level. So it is advised not to take caffeine after midday.

Excessive Sugar

Sugar can contribute to low energy levels, nervousness, sleep disturbance, and increased anxiety. Diet with a high amount of sugar easily zaps the energy level instead of boosting them. And at the same, it also increases your craving for a diet that is sugary, which takes you through the energy-draining circle.

Monosodium Glutamate (MSG)

This salt has been shown to affect most people by increasing their chances of getting an anxiety attack. How does it affect us? It does this by depleting the essential potassium in our system. Functionally, potassium is vital because it helps the nervous system to function properly, but monosodium glutamate uses the supply of potassium in the body. That increases blood pressure and strains the heart and arteries. This increased blood pressure can provoke the nervous system causing chest pain, headache, sleeplessness, and numbness, all of which are symptoms of anxiety. Their occurrence can even trigger an attack.

Alcohol

Alcohol can also worsen symptoms, and if it is used to self-medicate, it can lead to dependency issues. Alcohol changes the level of serotonin and other neurotransmitters in the brain, and that can worsen anxiety in an anxious person. In fact, a person with anxiety may feel more anxious after the alcohol wears off. This anxiety that returns after the alcohol wears off may last even longer.

Away from what to eat and what not to eat, let's look at other lifestyle changes that can be very efficient in the fight against anxiety disorders.

1. Exercise:

You must have heard that regular exercise is good for your health. Some people erroneously believe that health has to do with the physical body alone. But in the actual sense, a person is said to be healthy if they have a sound mind and body. So yes, exercising also improves the mind and helps relieve the illnesses that attack the mind, such as anxiety disorders. Exercise helps to relieve anxiety naturally because exercise is important for maintaining mental fitness, and it also helps reduce stress. It eases anxiety because it causes your body to release the feel-good hormones (endorphins), which lifts your mood. This is the reason why you feel elated just after exercising.

The best form of exercises for an anxiety disorder should be done as stipulated below:

- Aim for at least 30 minutes of aerobic exercise most days.
- Rhythmic activities that involve both arms and legs are effective—walking, running, swimming, dancing, etc.
- Maintaining a regular exercise routine associated with improved moves leads to better self-esteem and increased energy.

Such exercises can reduce the body's physical reaction to anxiety and the frequency/intensity of panic attacks. It can also help the body in releasing tension. Researchers have found that even a short brisk walk can provide several hours of relief. That is why physically active people have lower rates of anxiety than sedentary people. Exercise also helps the brain to cope with stress.

2. Stress reduction:

When we were discussing anxiety and panic disorders, we identified stress as one of the factors that can cause or contribute to those disorders. Since that is the case, it is only logical for you to look for a way to either eliminate the stress or manage it in such a way that it will not have too much impact on your mental health.

Chapter nine of this book will show you some stress management techniques that can help you cope with daily stressors that you cannot eliminate.

But before we discuss that, take a critical look at your daily routine today and start identifying those things that cause you stress. Once you have identified them, ask yourself, "can I eliminate this, or is it something I will have to put up with?" If you have to put up with it, see if there is a way you can reduce them. Oftentimes, there are ways you can cut down on those stressful tasks. For instance, look at your responsibilities and see if you can delegate them to others.

3. Sleep

I am sure you have heard that improper or insufficient sleep is harmful to your mind and body, but do you also know that lack of sleep can exacerbate anxious feelings? If you didn't know, well, now you do. The reason is that neurotransmitters that your body needs to support your moods are replenished when you are sleeping.

This is why you need to aim for 7–9 hours of quality sleep every night. I know that a lot is being said about hard workers who sacrifice their sleep for goals. You can work hard and achieve great things and still get sufficient sleep at night. It all boils down to efficient planning and timing.

And the fact that you have issues with anxiety further makes it very important for you of all people.

Research has found that people who deprive themselves of sleep are more likely to classify neutral images as negative. Everyday items can seem more menacing and contribute to anxiety. Anxiety can make it even more difficult for you to sleep.

If you're struggling to improve sleep quality or quantity, the following can help:

- Meditation.
- Exercise.
- Prioritization of to-do list.
- Listening to calming music.
- Removal of distractions such as turning off devices an hour before bed.
- Your sleeping environment should also be a calming space, with a moderated temperature of between 60 and 67 degrees Fahrenheit.
- Comfortable mattress and pillows make sleeping easier and better.

4. Social

If your anxiety isn't social anxiety disorder (SAD), this point will be lots easier for you. But if you are battling with SAD, chapter 5 will show you how you can manage to beat your fears and socialize more.

Loneliness and isolation can exacerbate anxiety symptoms because when you talk about your anxiety with people, this can make it less overwhelming. Try to see friends, relatives, coworkers, neighbors, and fellow worshippers whenever the need arises. Never shy away from it because if you do, you will be further validating the anxieties you have about yourself.

Another less socializing thing you can do is join support groups where you can hear from other people like you, and what they did or are doing to help their case. They could be your support network and look out for you when you are losing it.

You can also get yourself a lovely pet because your pet's company can help you too. Rather than focusing on yourself and your problems, you can focus your attention on caring for your pet and creating a great relationship with it.

In conclusion, all of the tips we have discussed in this chapter will only be effective if you quit chronic worrying. It is a mental habit that keeps you on edge every time. But the good news is that you can break it just like every other mental habit.

4

LIVING WITH GENERALIZED
ANXIETY DISORDER (GAD)

G AD is one of the most common anxiety disorders. It can significantly impact your life by creating emotional, behavioral, and physical symptoms. It is usual for someone to feel anxious sometimes. But it is a cause for concern if your fears and worries become constant and, as a result, hinder your body and soul from functioning and relaxing. Strategies to help you cope include social strategies, self-soothing, reframing your worries, and learning your triggers. While these approaches may not wholly cure GAD, they can make it much easier to live with.

GAD is diagnosed when your anxiety is so constant that it ends up interfering with your daily life. On more days than not, you may find it difficult to have control over worry for at least six months and have three or more of the symptoms discussed in this chapter.

Common anxiety disorders involve constant/chronic worrying, nervousness, and tension—not focused on one specific situation or thing. A person with a phobia has a fear that is connected to a particular thing or situation, which is entirely not the case with GAD. A person suffering from GAD has a diffused form of fear; they have a general feeling of unease that colours their whole life.

The anxiety related to GAD is usually less intense than a panic attack, but it tends to last longer. For panic attack, the feeling of fear occurs suddenly, and it is intense and tends to cause more harm to the person.

In the US, GAD affects 3.1% of the population and about 6.8 million adults in any given year. Women are twice as more susceptible to GAD than men. This type of anxiety comes on gradually and can begin across the life cycle. The risk is at its worst between childhood and middle age. The exact cause of GAD is unknown; however, there is evidence that family background, biological factors, and life experiences, especially stressful ones, plays a role.

A person with GAD may worry about similar things to other people but at a more intense level. For instance, a careless comment from a co-worker about the company's bad economy becomes a vision of imminent official notice that you have been fired from your job; a delayed response from a friend to a call or email leads to anxiety the relationship is coming to an end. Most times, even the thought of getting through the day develops anxiety. People with GAD have a form of exaggerated worry or tension as they go about their activities. This is the case even when there is little or nothing to worry about. They find it very difficult or even impossible to turn off their anxious thoughts, even when they know that their anxiety or worry is more intense than the situation warrants and try to stop it. They usually think this worry is beyond their control.

People with GAD, whose anxiety level is mild to moderate or with treatment, can have full and meaningful lives, be gainfully employed, and function socially. But people with GAD must avoid situations that may trigger anxiety. They should try not to take advantage of opportunities due to their worry (travel, promotions, social situations, etc.). Many have trouble carrying out the simplest daily activities when their anxiety level is high.

THE DIFFERENCE BETWEEN GAD AND "NORMAL" WORRY

It is a normal part of life for you to have doubts, worries, and fears. It is also natural to be anxious about a future event or situation, such as an upcoming exam, or a delayed funds transaction into your account. The difference between GAD and "normal" worrying is that the worries emanated from

GAD are usually excessive, disruptive, persistent, and intrusive.

The difference between Generalized Anxiety Disorder (GAD) and "Normal" Worry

Generalized Anxiety Disorder:	"Normal" Worry
It hinders your activities, job, or social life.	It doesn't hinder your daily responsibilities and activities.
It is uncontrollable	It is controllable
It is extremely stressful and upsetting.	It may be unpleasant, but it doesn't lead to significant distress.
It emanates from all sorts of things, expecting the worst from each.	It is limited to a particular, small case of realistic concerns.
This form of worry exists for at least six months. almost	This form of worry lasts for only a short period of time.

SYMPTOMS OF GENERALIZED ANXIETY DISORDER (GAD)

The symptoms of GAD can differ from person to person depending on several factors such as biological factors, and life experiences. In this section of our investigation of living with GAD, we will discuss the emotional, behavioral, and physical symptoms of GAD.

Emotional:

- You are constantly worried about things and situations, even about the situations beyond your control and those that don't call for worry. The worrying associated with GAD is disproportionate to the situations that trigger it.

- Over time, you will develop a feeling that your anxiety is uncontrollable, and may end up giving in to it by concluding that there is nothing you can do to prevent or stop the worrying.

- Most often, you are faced with intrusive thoughts about the things and situations that make you anxious. Although you may try to stop thinking about them, you can't.

- You have an inability to tolerate uncertainty; you feel you need to know what is going to happen beforehand.

- A pervasive feeling of apprehension always confronts you.

Behavioral

- You are always unable to relax, be by yourself, or enjoy the quiet time because you are confronted by a sense of impending danger, doom, or panic. Although restlessness doesn't occur in all people with GAD, it is one of the red flags doctors frequently look out for during diagnosis. If you experienced restlessness frequently for longer than six months, it might be a sign of GAD.

- Many people with GAD complain about having difficulty concentrating. However, difficulty concentrating is also related to other medical conditions such as depression, so it is not enough evidence to diagnose GAD.
- You always want to put things off because you feel overwhelmed.
- You tend to avoid several situations because they make you anxious.

Physical

- Having tense muscles on most days is another report that doctors look for during diagnosis because it's a common symptom associated with GAD. It is possible that GAD leads to increased muscle tenseness, but it is also possible that muscle tenseness leads to increased GAD, or that a third factor causes both.
- Difficulty falling/staying asleep is strongly associated with anxiety disorders. Many people with GAD report that they wake up in the middle of the night and have difficulty falling asleep. Some research shows that having insomnia during childhood is linked to developing GAD later in life. Insomnia and anxiety are strongly linked but it is

unclear whether anxiety contributes to insomnia, if insomnia contributes to anxiety, or both. However, it has been observed that when a general anxiety disorder is treated, insomnia often improves as well.

- Most people with GAD feel excessive restlessness or irritability.

According to a recent study on over 6,000 adults, it was observed that more than 90% of those with GAD reported feeling irritable, especially when their anxiety level was at its peak.

Young and middle-aged adults with GAD reported twice as much irritability in their daily routine.

- Stomach problems, diarrhea, or nausea are some red flag symptoms associated with GAD.

GAD symptoms in children

Excessive worrying in children centers on past behaviors, future events, family matters, social acceptance, personal abilities, and school performance. Unlike adults with this anxiety disorder, children and teens often don't realize that their anxiety is disproportionate to the event or situation, so adults need to recognize their symptoms. In addition to the many symptoms that appear in adults discussed above, some red flags for GAD in children are:

- "What if" fears; a child with GAD may become so worried about situations far in the future, most of which are beyond their control.
- Perfectionism; you may begin to notice the fear of making mistakes and excessive self-criticism in the behavior of your child.
- Many children with GAD feel that they are to blame for any disaster that may occur, and their worry will keep tragedy from occurring.
- The strong belief that misfortune is contagious and will happen to them in the future. This conviction leads to an anxiety disorder.
- Children with GAD need frequent reassurance and approval because they feel less confident in their abilities and capabilities.

SOCIAL COPING STRATEGIES

When we have GAD, it is common to want to disconnect from others and isolate ourselves. This feeling of loneliness even increases our anxiety. For some people, social strategies can help to manage symptoms and is a vital means to overcome GAD. For instance, going out to watch your favorite games will keep your mind focused on the fun of the game, therefore, keeping every form of anxiety at bay. Below are some social coping strategies to manage your anxiety.

Participating in social activities can make you feel less alone and can also provide a distraction that makes you forget the cause of your impending anxiety.

It is very important that you find someone you can always talk to because talking to someone about your anxiety can make you feel less alone. This is particularly helpful when your worries start spiraling. You could also talk to a specialist on anxiety control.

When you are struggling with anxiety, social activities help you to find a support system. Support groups can provide you with a network of people going through the same thing. There are a variety of support groups available, both online and in-person options, that can be of great significance when it comes to managing GAD.

Anxiety tends to rob us of pleasure and hinders us from having the fun we deserve. Laughter can help alleviate symptoms, and this can be found through friends and family. You can also find humor on television, in books, or online sources.

Know who to avoid when your anxiety is high. Other people who worry may not be helpful at this time; also, people you know tend to stress you out.

Be aware that your anxiety may get in the way of your relationships at times, leaving you feeling needy and insecure.

Look for anxiety-driven relationship patterns and take steps to reduce them. It is possible that each time you are with someone undesirable, your anxiety level keeps increasing. It is advisable you figure what relationships are and how you can put an end to them.

STRATEGIES TO HELP YOU CALM DOWN QUICKLY

Social Interaction.

Social interaction can help you calm down quickly, but when this isn't possible, you can self-soothe using physical senses:

- Sight: look at things that relax you or make you smile. If you can't go out for a recreational view of tourism centers, you could entertain your sight with family pictures, pets' pictures from the internet, or television.
- Sound: listen to soothing sounds or music or create music with musical Instruments. You could sing

your favorite tune or listen to the sounds of nature (either live or recorded), the wind through the trees, ocean waves, or birds singing.

- Smell: you can also manage your anxiety by lighting scented candles, spraying on your favorite perfume, and breathing in fresh air.
- Taste: having a good taste of your favorite treat will help reduce your anxiety. You could also use a sip of herbal tea as it will also help.
- Touch: self-massage, stroke a pet, stroke a soft blanket, or sitting outside in the cool breeze are very good ways to help you manage GAD.
- Movement: walking around with a friend or pet, jumping up and down and stretching your joints, and dancing are very good ways to manage anxiety.

Reframing Your Worries

The major symptom of GAD is excessive worrying, which is derived from your internal beliefs. You may feel your worries come from external factors, but worrying is self-generated. The trigger is external, but it is your internal dialogue that feeds it.

You probably try to solve problems that haven't happened yet and predict worst-case scenarios. This may feel like self-protection, but it's causing the problem. To save yourself from the psychological stress of anxiety, you have to stop assuming the worst in every upcoming event. You have to develop a sense of optimism. Visualize the event coming to pass in the best possible manner. Don't forget that you may be worrying yourself for an event that may finally happen in your favor.

Try to stop focusing on "what if's." You probably have a lot of "what if's" running through your head. This increases your heartbeat and anxiety level. To avoid making your GAD worse, you have to stop visualizing upcoming events, especially those that make you uncomfortable. Those worst-case events you have imagined have less than 10% chance of actually happening. Is that worth the stress? Hell no. You are obviously paying in advance for a commodity you may likely not get delivered.

Some people with GAD actually think worrying will help them salvage the effects of the unlikely event they have visualized. Let go of the idea that worrying helps you because it doesn't. As a matter of fact, worrying causes more harm to your health.

Challenge Worrisome Thoughts:

Create a daily worry period: To have absolute control over your worries, you have to set time and place for worrying, for instance, in the bathroom from 6:00 to 6:20 pm. You have to ensure your preferred worry period comes way before your bedtime. During this period, you are free to worry about whatever is in your mind.

Distinguish between solvable and unsolvable worries: Problem-solving has to do with evaluating a situation and figuring out concrete steps to remedy the situation. Taking your time to think about the worst-case scenario is never the solution to any upcoming situation. Instead, you need to figure out if your worry is solvable or not. If your worry is actually solvable, you need to spend more time brainstorming on the possible remedies. But if your worry is not solvable, you have to accept the uncertainty.

Interrupt the worry cycle: The thoughts associated with GAD usually come like a boomerang. You have to interrupt the worry circle to give yourself a time out of the excessive and relentless worrying. To do this, you have to engage in one or more of the following:

1. Get up and get moving by engaging in some exercises. They release endorphins that boost energy, relieve stress, and enhance your sense of welfare.
2. Take a tai chi or yoga class. Basically, this has to do with focusing your mind on your breathing and movements.

3. Meditate. This helps in switching your focus from the past or future to what's happening in the present.

4. Try deep breathing. Worrying increases the rate of your breathing, which increases your anxiety. To take control of your breath and quiet negative thoughts associated with anxiety, you have to practice deep breathing.

Practice Mindfulness

Anxiety is basically worrying about what might take place in the future and what you will do about it. Sometimes it has to do with past events, rehashing the things you have done or said. Mindfulness helps you reduce your worries by conveying your attention to the present each time you get overwhelmed by your worries. With mindfulness, you can figure out where your thinking is doing you damage, and get in touch with your emotions. You have to acknowledge and observe your worries, and not try to fight, ignore, or control them. After figuring out and accepting your worries, you have to let them go. Try as much as you can to always stay focused in the present by paying attention to how your body feels, your ever-changing emotions, the rhythm of your breathing, and the thoughts that drift through your mind. We will discuss more about mindfulness in chapter eight.

.   .   .

Practice Relaxation Techniques

The meditation techniques can provide some immediate respite from anxiety and worry. These relaxation techniques will also change your brain if practiced regularly. It will be further discussed in chapter nine.

Learn Your Triggers

In as much as you seek to manage your anxiety, it is also important you pay attention to the things, events, or situations that seem to trigger your anxiety. It may not be easy to avoid those triggers completely, but knowing them will go a long way to helping you gain clarity and enable you to take steps to manage stress in those specific situations.

Practice Acceptance

You don't have to feel bad if you are experiencing anxiety. It is not something you are facing because you are flawed in any way. It is influenced by a number of factors. GAD is something that many people experience, and there is no one cause for it.

Adopt A Positive Attitude

It is important you keep a positive attitude when experiencing GAD. You don't have to lose hope for better living because of GAD. Many people challenged by anxiety live full, joyful, and productive lives. I will recommend some inspiration through verses, quotes, nature, music, and social connections, etc.

Generally, GAD can be a disturbing condition to have, but it is not a death sentence. If you can discipline yourself to follow the tips we have discussed and will still discuss, you will cope with your symptoms and live your best life.

5

LIVING WITH SOCIAL ANXIETY DISORDER

When people give speeches, they experience anxiety. Even the most celebrated orators get this anxiety. The difference between good speakers and people who fumble is that the good speakers know how to conceal their anxiety and proceed with the task as if they are not anxious. If you are one of these bold speakers who don't experience anxiety when you speak, it could be that you get your social anxiety when you are attending an interview. We all do, but to different degrees.

It is not just during speeches or interviews that people get anxious. Many people experience some degree of anxiety in social situations such as parties, schools, dates, and other human-to-human interactions. When moderate, it can be considered normal. But when this anxiety becomes intense and interferes with your life, you may be experiencing social anxiety disorder (SAD), which comes with emotional, behavioral, and physical symptoms and can be very distressing.

As I said in the preliminary chapters of this book, SAD is one of the main types of anxiety disorders. And in this chapter, we will take an in-depth look at this disorder. We will look at the signs and symptoms, thinking styles that fuel it, and self-help, among other things.

WHAT IS SAD?

We know how people can be shy or develop occasional nerves when they are in public, but SAD is more than regular shyness. It is a condition whereby an individual develops an intense fear for certain social situations. The fear can be more intense when the individual is confronting a social situation that they are not familiar with. The fear stems from the erroneous belief that the individual is being watched and evaluated by others. That, most times, is not the case because most times, people are too busy living their own lives that they won't have the spare time to start assessing you.

There is a difference between social anxiety and social anxiety disorder. You need to know the underlying difference. You can get anxious during a social setting. If it starts and ends with that social setting and doesn't linger or try to interfere with your life decisions after that situation, it is just social anxiety. But if you get the anxiety and, because of it, you decide you are never going to be in that setting or anything similar, it is becoming a disorder. If you also catch yourself getting anxious just by thinking of that social setting, then it is a disorder. In a nutshell, you may experience social anxiety in some situations without having SAD. But when your anxiety affects your life and causes great stress, it may be SAD.

People with SAD do not just stop at believing they are being evaluated; they also believe that people's evaluation of them will be negative. Since they are scared that they might be scrutinized, judged or, maybe even embarrassed, they may go to great lengths to avoid these situations. They will do everything to avoid that situation because they don't want to be embarrassed. And even when they just think about those social situations, they may become anxious.

The problem with such avoidance is that you land out avoiding things that are fun and exhilarating for others, such as parties with friends, hangouts, graduation ceremonies, and so on. Apart from that, it can keep you from reaching great heights in your chosen career. That is because you will do everything to avoid assessments such as interviews and examinations. And even when you force yourself to attend because you badly need to do so, you might end up ruining everything because your panic will get the better part of you. Even if you are already working, you try to avoid those presentations and interactions that can grant you promotions and growth in your workplace.

SAD also reduces your confidence and can give you chronic low self-esteem that will force you not to try anything because you have convinced yourself that you are not good enough. In extreme cases, it can spiral into depression, and if not attended to, can lead to isolation, or worst-case scenario, suicide.

So you can see that this is not a disorder you want to live with. If you hadn't realized that you are living with SAD all this while, that is pardonable. Now that you know, you must do everything you can to emancipate yourself from such mental slavery.

If this describes you, all hope is not lost. There are a few proven tips that you can start using today to reclaim your confidence and mingle with people healthily.

CAUSES AND COMMON

If you have SAD, you are not alone; countless other people are with you. Anxiety and Depression Association of America (ADAA) states that, in the U.S., around 40 million people experience one form of anxiety every year, and out of that number, 15 million of them experience social anxiety. SAD is quite common, but different things can cause it in different people.

Common triggers include:

- Meeting new people: If you have SAD, then you know how difficult it is for you to strike up a conversation with a total stranger. That is because you feel that you do not deserve their time, and they shouldn't be talking to you. This is the same reason why you might find it difficult to go on a date. For people with SAD, being on a date or thinking about one can trigger anxiety.

- Small talk: For people with SAD, small talk is not just a mutual communication between pairs; they see it as an evaluation exercise. They start picking their words and being careful. This can lead to a slight mistake in speech, and when that happens, they spiral out of control, and anxiety sets in.

- Public speaking: Even people who do not have anxiety disorders get anxious when speaking in public, and they know it is normal. It doesn't stop them from speaking in public because they understand it is normal. In contrast, people with SAD experience anxiety once, and decide they will never do it again because of how they felt about it the first time. They make it all about themselves and assume that their listeners are there to evaluate them when, in reality, they are there to hear or even learn from them.

Other triggers include:

- Stage performance
- Being the center of attention
- Being watched
- Being teased
- Going on a date
- Talking to authority figures
- Speaking in a meeting
- Using public bathrooms
- Taking exams
- Making phone calls
- Going to parties

Basically, any situation that can make you believe that you are being evaluated can make you anxious if you live with SAD. By that, you will start seeing that situation as a psychologically stressful situation, and you will do anything you can to avoid it. As you start avoiding it, it begins to disrupt your life, and that is when it goes from an annoying situation to a disorder.

SYMPTOMS OF SAD

Symptoms are the subtle or extreme signs that you can use to tell for sure that you are grappling with SAD. Most people live in denial; they like to tell themselves that it is probably normal because they know that every one of us gets anxious.

Being anxious is okay, just as we saw in the first chapter of this book, but when it goes beyond mere anxiety, and you start noticing the following symptoms, you may have SAD.

The symptoms can be divided into emotional, behavioral, and physical.

1. Emotional symptoms: These are the feelings you will get because of the anxiety you feel.

- Excessive self-consciousness.
- Intense worry leading up to a social situation (sometimes months in advance)
- Extreme fear of being judged
- Fear that you'll embarrass yourself
- Fear that others will notice your anxiety

2. Behavioral symptoms: These are some of the behaviors you would put up that you probably wouldn't have if you weren't concerned about people's evaluation of you.

- Avoiding social situations
- Staying quiet and trying to go unnoticed
- Need to bring someone with you
- Drinking before social situations

3. Physical symptoms: These are the ways your physical body will react to the anxiety you are feeling on the inside.

- Blushing
- Shortness of breath
- Stomach upset
- Trembling/shaking
- Racing heart
- Sweating
- Feeling faint

STRATEGIES FOR OVERCOMING SAD

There are several strategies you can adopt to help you deal with this, although they all involve you facing social situations head-on. Just because it involves facing the situation headlong, most people with SAD will prefer not even to try, but that is not you. Just the fact that you are reading this book shows you want to be free. You have to follow this through to reach that freedom.

For you, it will get as easy as it can get because, in this chapter, you will see how misplaced those fears are. When you have learned to see your fears as lacking basis, you will find it easier to face the situations on your way to recovery.

Avoid Negative Coping Strategies

Most people, when they discover that they feel overly anxious about certain social settings, get creative and start looking for things that can help them cope with those settings, especially when it is inevitable. ADAA's statistics that state that 20% of people with SAD also have alcohol use disorder proves this assertion. That would have been great, but the problem is that most of these coping strategies will only harm you in the long run because you have not faced the problem squarely. The most common coping strategy that people adopt is alcohol and substance consumption. Another problem with this is that it can lead to substance dependence and abuse. For instance, if you start taking alcohol to help you get over your panic so that you can address your coworkers at work, you will never be able to address anyone when you are sober. With time, you may become an alcoholic, and that, on its own, has its own demerits.

Also, when you take too much of these substances, it can even worsen your anxiety and lead to further isolation. Research shows that excessive drinking can circle back and cause heightened anxiety, bad moods, and other symptoms such as disrupted sleep patterns. So avoid negative coping strategies by all means. If you have started using them already, stop. Remember that a healthy lifestyle can help you cope with most of the anxiety disorders, and in the third chapter of this book, we said a healthy lifestyle also entails cutting down on alcohol.

Face Your Fear

Rather than looking to hide behind alcohol or other substances, learn to face these situations with sobriety because you will be sober most of the time. And it is only when you have conquered it with your clear eyes that you have truly conquered it. Not everyone will take substances to mask their anxiety. Instead, they will slip into isolation because they want to avoid engaging in social situations as much as they can.

In this era that we live in, isolation is even easier for them because of the internet, smartphones, and social media. People prefer to attend online events and keep ghost friends because they don't want physical contact. As people hide behind their smartphones and become addicted to technology, they begin to display potential markers of social anxiety.

Facing your fear is a therapeutic approach that works because it violates your norms and standards to break the self-reinforcing cycle of fear and avoidance. When you expose yourself to social mishaps, those social settings you are scared of, you gradually begin to see how baseless your fears are. You will realize that instead of your listeners judging you and embarrassing you as you anticipated, they may even give you a standing ovation. You will realize that your perceived threats do not lead to the negative consequences you had conjured in your mind. That will force you to reevaluate the perceived threats.

In essence, that social setting that you dread most should dominate your to-do list. If you dread public speaking, look to snatch every opportunity that comes your way to address people. Do this continually, and it becomes easier.

Reframe Your Thoughts

You have seen how most of the negative consequences that you have framed up are mostly false. It is a thing of the mind because you are what you tell yourself. If you tell yourself that you are not good enough for human interaction, you will live your life believing that. But suppose you tell yourself that you are the best version of you. In that case, you will see yourself as worthy of associating with other people without expecting to be evaluated negatively. Hence, you must learn to reframe your thoughts on how you understand the stress you are experiencing.

Learn to focus on an affirming thought that can make it easier to deal with a social situation. For instance, even if attending a party seems like a daunting task, tell yourself, "the party is scary, but I am a funny and interesting person, so I should blend in just fine because I will have talking points with people I encounter."

It is recommended that for the best result, you should counter each of your negative thoughts with at least three positive ones.

Perform An Act Of Kindness

When you do this, it can help counter negative social expectations by forming an association of positivity with the social environment. The act of kindness can also distract you from focusing on yourself too much, worrying, and conjuring negative thoughts about yourself. Apart from distracting you, kind deeds also have a way of lifting moods and making you happier. Countless research agrees so.

For these reasons, selfless acts of kindness can help people with SAD to feel better in social situations, and one study published in Motivation and Emotion in 2015 agrees.

. . .

Challenge Negative Thoughts

Before you can reframe your thoughts, you have to eliminate the negative thoughts, and one way you can do that is by challenging them.

- Identify negative thoughts: For instance, you may have told yourself that you are not as good as others. That is a negative thought.
- Analyze and challenge the thought: What are your reasons for saying this? Are you created differently than others? What are your reasons for coming up with such a drastic conclusion?
- Logical evaluation: As you begin to pick sentiments apart and evaluate everything logically, it can help you replace these thoughts with more positive and realistic ones.

Unhealthy Thinking Styles

Unhealthy thinking styles can fuel social anxiety. Look for unhelpful thought styles you may be having such as:

- Mind reading: A situation where you will assume that you know what other people are thinking. When you assume this, you will also assume that they see you in the same negative light that you see yourself.

- Fortune telling: When you try to predict the future and foretelling doom for yourself. Beliefs like "If I stand up to talk, I will embarrass myself." When did you start knowing the future?
- Catastrophizing: Exaggerating things more than what they are. For instance, believing that people will notice that you are anxious, and it will be terrible.
- Personalizing: Making everything all about you and assuming that people see you negatively.

Learn to Focus On Other People Rather Than Yourself

It is when you overthink yourself and about people's evaluation of you that anxiety kicks in. Focusing on yourself and how you're feeling in the situation triggers more anxiety and prevents you from being present in the social situation. Learn to shift your attention to others. The more you concentrate on what's happening around you, the less you'll be affected by anxiety.

As you focus on other people, don't try to imagine what they are thinking about you, remember that is what we are trying to avoid.

Here are a few tips to further help you overcome your SAD.

- Remember that your anxiety isn't that visible, so people will be concerned with their affairs rather than judging you.
- Keep your focus on the social setting and listen to what's being said.
- Focus on the present.
- Stop pressuring yourself to be perfect. We are all humans, and we are not perfect. Rather than worrying about your imperfection, channel that energy into improving that aspect of your life if it is possible. But if you can't improve on it, accept it as a part of you and learn to live with it,
- Control your breathing in a social situation. We will be discussing more on controlled breathing when we start discussing more detailed self-care methods for anxiety disorders.
- Make an effort to be more social. SAD wants you to be in isolation, but you know you must not yield to it. So strive to be more social against all the odds.
- Look for supportive social environments that are not focused on socializing, such as classes and voluntary work.
- Practice assertiveness.
- Work on non-verbal communication skills. These

are skills that can make you more confident in social interactions. It involves knowing how to take a relaxed posture because that can encourage people to respond positively to you. Ordinarily, SAD causes you to have a "closed-off" stance that tends to scare people away and reinforce your fear.

- Improve communication skills: When you know how to communicate effectively, you will find it easier to socialize, and you will rarely make those mistakes that can hurt your self-esteem and sink you.

- Be open about your anxiety; talk about it. As you talk about it, you will begin to see how senseless it sounds. Your listener can also help you debunk some of the erroneous beliefs you have about yourself.

Everyday Strategies

- Inform your employer.
- Arrive at meetings/appointments early.
- List questions before an event.
- Keep up with current events to give fodder for small talk.
- Attend events/do a job where you derive true value, so the social elements seem worth it.

- Aim to make new friends.
- Practice healthy lifestyle habits that we discussed in the third chapter of this book.

Above all, remember that social anxiety is not a personality trait, meaning that it does not come naturally as your way of thinking, feeling, and behaving. Therefore, you can work on it.

In conclusion, it can be extremely difficult living with SAD or trying to free yourself from it, but it is possible to set yourself free. You can start by challenging the negative thoughts that trigger your fear and anxiety. Then proceed to face your fears by facing the situations that give you sleepless nights. As you expose yourself to those situations you dread so much, and you realize that they are not as embarrassing as you thought, you will find it easier to face them a second time. It will teach you to stay anxiety-free in those situations you consider stressful. If you practice the self-care approaches we've discussed here, you should do just fine. But if you think you may need extra care and attention, consult a doctor or other mental health professionals.

6

LIVING WITH OBSESSIVE-COMPULSIVE DISORDER

O CD is yet another common anxiety disorder. Here is a guide to understanding it, its symptoms, triggers, types, diagnosis, risk factors, and some self-care steps that you can adopt today if you have this disorder.

A person might lock the door to their apartment on their way out, and a few meters away from the door, they feel a strong urge to double-check that they locked the door. The person in this context had a genuine reason for double-checking. They simply wanted to be sure their home was secured. They wanted to do it, and they did it. In the case of somebody with OCD, the person in this example will lock the door, know very well that they locked it, yet they will feel a strong compulsion to go and check again. Deep down, they know they locked the door, but the compulsion will get a better part of them. And they will return to check the door even when they know they did. They went back to check the door even when it complicates their life unnecessarily.

WHAT IS OCD?

It is an anxiety disorder characterized by a cycle of obsessions and compulsions, which can be difficult to prevent. If you have OCD, you will normally experience repetitive and unwanted thoughts that lead to excessive urges to do the things that dominate your thoughts. These thoughts are known as obsessions, while excessive urges are known as compulsions. These obsessive thoughts and compulsive behaviors can interfere with your life. When they do, you have OCD.

To better understand OCD, let's look at the obsession and compulsion components individually.

Obsessions: They are thoughts, images, and impulses that recur. They are often disturbing and distracting to you, and they are repetitive.

Compulsions: They are behaviors/rituals that you feel compelled to act out repeatedly, usually as an attempt to reduce obsessions (e.g., fear of contamination = cleaning rituals). But relief does not last, and the obsessions often come back stronger, and the rituals only add to anxiety.

OCD is an anxiety disorder because even when you know that your thoughts and behaviors are illogical, you will still be worried and anxious that if you don't do them, something terrible might happen. Whenever you try to ignore or suppress these thoughts, you will be afraid that the thoughts you are having might just be true. It is when this anxiety becomes too much that you will eventually cave in and engage in those compulsive behaviors. When you engage in the behavior, your anxiety reduces, but only temporarily. Soon, the obsessive thoughts will be on to you again.

With OCD, you are trapped in a cyclical pattern of obsessive thoughts to anxiety to compulsive behavior to temporary relief. When the relief wears off, the obsessive thoughts resume.

While it is possible for some people to experience either obsession or compulsion, others experience obsessions and compulsions together, and that is when it is said that they have OCD.

When you have OCD, obsessive thoughts and compulsive behaviors interfere with your everyday life. It is characterized by uncontrollable, unwanted thoughts and ritualized behaviors you feel compelled to perform; you may know they're irrational, but you cannot resist them. You may have obsessive thoughts and behave compulsively, and it will not qualify as a disorder. However, whenever these obsessions and compulsions become so distressing that they affect your life, it becomes a disorder.

The brain gets stuck on a thought or urge, which can only be relieved by performing repetitive behaviors.

RISK FACTORS

It has been stated that genetics play a role in OCD. That means that you are more likely to develop it if a biological relative has it.

Most times, OCD doesn't occur alone. It often co-occurs with Attention Deficit Hyperactivity Disorder (ADHD), Tourette's, major depressive disorder, social anxiety disorder, and eating disorders.

The symptoms associated with OCD are often exacerbated by stress.

CATEGORIES OF PEOPLE WITH OCD

People with OCD fall into categories of:

- Washers: these are people who are afraid of contamination. They are characterized by washing compulsions. For instance, you may find yourself washing your hand twenty times before touching a food item because you fear that you may contaminate that food if you don't wash that way.

- Checkers: these people will check something time and time again because they feel that if they don't, they may be exposed to harm or danger. For instance, a checker may visit the kitchen several times, and each time, they check that they turned off the gas cooker because they don't want to burn down the house.

- Doubters and sinners: this category of people have a strong belief that if they fail to do things perfectly, something terrible will happen to them.

- Counters and arrangers: these people's obsessions are with order and symmetry. They are driven by superstitions about numbers, order, colors, and other symmetry-related items. A counter/arranger will spend time checking that a group of items is arranged in a particular manner because they dread something bad will happen if these are not arranged "properly."

- Hoarders: these people are scared that if they dispose of anything, then something bad will happen to them. That will cause them to compulsively keep things even when they don't need it. Hoarders may also suffer from other related mental illnesses such as PTSD, kleptomania,

ADHD, skin picking, depression, compulsive buying, and tic disorders.

SYMPTOMS OF OCD

Symptoms can express themselves through thoughts and behaviors.

Thoughts: The common ones are:

- Fear of contamination
- Fear of harming yourself or others
- Intrusive sexual or violent thoughts
- Excessive focus on religious/moral concepts
- Fear of not having things you may need
- Order and symmetry
- Superstitions

Behaviors: The common behaviors you will notice yourself exhibiting are:

- Excessive checking of objects
- Repeatedly checking on loved ones
- counting/tapping/repeating certain words
- Excessive washing/cleaning
- Ordering and arranging things
- Excessive prayer

- Accumulating junk

COPING STRATEGIES/ SELF-CARE TIPS

Identifying your triggers, practicing exposure and response prevention (ERP), and challenging negative thoughts can help you to manage your condition, as well as making lifestyle changes and adopting techniques that can help with all kinds of anxiety disorders, such as relaxation and meditation techniques.

In the case of OCD, and just about any anxiety disorder that we are discussing so far, I don't need to stress the importance of learning all you can about the condition you have. This is the best way to confront it. Reading this book is a great place to start, but it shouldn't be the last. Learn as much as you can about any of the disorders you have. Without that, your anxiety is higher when you don't have any idea of what is happening to you. Strive to become an expert on your condition, then proceed with the following self-help tips:

Identify your triggers

This is the first step to managing OCD. Your triggers are those thoughts or situations that initiate the obsessions and compulsions. To identify your trigger also means recording it. If something happens and it leads to an obsession, record what happened, and the obsession it led to. Also, record the intensity of the anxiety that ensued and the compulsions that you used to ease the anxiety. For instance, if you are a washer, touching a contaminated substance may trigger an intense fear that you have been contaminated, and you may have to wash your hands for several minutes before you eased the anxiety that followed. In this case, the trigger was the dirty substance. Give the fear or anxiety you felt a number on a scale of one to ten. Then record the number of times you had to wash your hands before the anxiety died down.

Why is this important? When you keep track of triggers, you may be able to anticipate your obsessions. And if you can anticipate them, you will be able to appease them more easily. For instance, if you know that you are a washer, take extra care to wash the first time so that when the urge comes for you to wash again, you know it is a compulsion. Another example is if you are a checker, tempted to check and double-check that you locked the door, pay more attention the first time you locked it.

As you lock the door the first time, create a clear and solid mental picture at the back of your mind that tells you that you locked the door for sure. When you do that, and the urge comes for you to check the door again, you will quickly identify this new wave of urge for what it is: nothing but an obsessive thought.

This routine can help you ease the anxiety that follows. It can also serve as an important tool for you to start learning how to handle other OCD compulsions because as you proceed with one, you will begin to see a pattern that works.

Learn to resist compulsions

You may say, "If I identify my triggers, is it not better to avoid the situations altogether?" That might seem like a good idea, but you have to realize that the more you avoid those triggers, the scarier they get. So instead of avoiding, learn to resist them by exposing yourself to them. Remember how we said in the previous chapter that it was better to expose yourself to the social settings that scare you if you have SAD. Here, too, it is better to expose yourself to your triggers so that, with time, they will no longer be scary.

Exposing yourself to the trigger and learning how to deal with the anxiety without giving in to the urges is how you get over OCD. This technique is called the exposure and response prevention (ERP) technique. Qualified mental health experts use this technique when offering therapy to their patients.

With ERP, you go to where the trigger or source of your obsession is, then you stop yourself from performing the compulsive behavior that would have eased your anxiety. For instance, if you are a washer and you will go to a public restroom, you have to touch the door handle. Normally, this was enough to get you washing and washing again, but this time, keep yourself from washing at all. The anxiety will hit you, but choose to sit this one out. With time, the anxiety will begin to go, and you will realize, much to your amazement, that the anxiety can go away even when you don't give in to your obsession.

It is not going to be the easiest thing you will do, so don't expect an easy ride. The difficulty that comes with it is the reason why you should start with your smallest fears first and move up. Remember that while you were identifying your triggers, you were attaching numbers to them according to their intensity. When you want to start confronting your fears, start with those with a lower intensity number. Arrange your fears in ascending order of intensity and work your way up the ladder.

Challenge obsessive thoughts

We all get troubling thoughts from time to time, and that's normal. But with OCD, your brain is stuck on a particular recurring anxiety-provoking thought. The more distressing the thought is to you, the more you will try to repress it. This attempt to repress it will only cause it to become more bothersome. As with compulsions, you can train yourself with ERP. Remind yourself that your thoughts do not define you; no matter how violent or intrusive they are, they don't make you a bad person. To see your thoughts for what they truly are, do the following:

- Write down your obsessive thoughts. No matter how repetitive it gets, write it down. Doing this will make it lose its power. Also, writing it down is harder than just thinking about them, so it helps your obsessive thoughts to disappear sooner.

- Create an OCD worry period. Schedule specific times to focus on these thoughts. Rather than allowing these thoughts to meddle in your day, set time aside when you can accommodate those worries. I recommend ten minutes each day. During this time, you are focusing on these thoughts but not trying to correct them. After the period, calm yourself and let the thoughts go so you can focus on living your life for the rest of the day. When obsessive thoughts come into your mind, rather than worrying about them, write them down and postpone them to your worry period.

- Challenge the thoughts. Ask yourself, "Is this thought I am having now helpful?" "Are there more positive or realistic views of the situation?" "Is there any evidence that the thought is true, and if there is, what is it?" "If a friend was having this same thought, what would I say to them?"

- Record yourself saying the thought out loud and expose yourself to it regularly to reduce distress.

Find Support

If you have OCD, look to create a support network such as OCD support groups, friends, and family for yourself. This is because OCD can consume you and push you to isolation. And if you give in to isolation, it will only worsen your OCD symptoms, so you must never let it get to that. How can you do that? Through support. Create time for your family and friends. Locate and join OCD groups so you can learn from people's experiences and find support when you will need it.

Manage stress

Try to minimize stress as much as possible because it can trigger symptoms and also aggravate your OCD. You can reduce stress by exercising regularly and spending time with the people who matter in your life. You can also adopt the relaxation techniques we will be discussing later in this book.

Make lifestyle changes:

This has been discussed extensively in chapter three. With OCD, you need to get enough sleep, eat well, exercise regularly, meditate, and stick with your treatment plan.

- Practice mindfulness: We will discuss more on this in chapter eight.
- Practice relaxation techniques: Refer to chapter nine.
- Become informed about OCD: The more you know about the condition, the better equipped you are to handle it. Also, educating yourself in OCD will expose you to support networks and other people facing similar problems. By reading this book, you have set yourself on the right track. You can still know more about the condition by reading online books and contents on it. You can also talk to your mental wellness experts or doctors if you need any help or information.

In conclusion, treatment of OCD can be done through consultation with a qualified mental health expert who will prescribe medications. Still, these self-help strategies are just as good, if not better, because they help you attack the problem from the roots, and not just improve the symptoms as medication would.

7

THE POWER OF EFT TAPPING IN MANAGING ANXIETY

I know how challenging dealing with anxiety can be. However, on the bright side, there are many effective coping strategies you can use. I have explained the three most common forms of anxiety disorder in the previous sections. By now, you should know that there are some techniques you can use to manage your anxiety, whether it has become a disorder or not. Whether you are aware or not, it is important to know and also identify the type that works for you to help you manage your symptoms while living with the condition.

Exercise, meditation, therapy, and lifestyle changes, among other things, are all wonderful ways that you can use to relieve your symptoms. If you are already practicing any of them, I commend you, because you are already putting in the effort and taking an active role in improving your health and wellbeing.

But again, you may be practicing all these and still suffering from anxiety symptoms. In that case, what should you do?

This is where Tapping comes in. Tapping is a technique that helps in managing anxiety.

WHAT IS EFT TAPPING?

The emotional freedom technique (EFT) was developed by Gary Craig in 1993. It is a form of alternative medicine that is similar to acupuncture. Although Tapping is something that you can do for yourself, you don't need help from someone like you do with acupuncture.

There is ongoing research into EFT. Still, it has been suggested as an effective way to manage anxiety and PTSD. Since it's still undergoing research, it would be best when used with other techniques for managing anxiety.

Simply put, EFT, also referred to as Tapping or psychological acupuncture, is an alternative treatment for emotional distress.

HOW EFT TAPPING WORKS

The basis of science on Tapping therapy borders on the functions of the amygdala. The amygdala is an almond-shaped part of the human brain. It is part of your limbic system and serves as a source of long-term memory and emotions.

The amygdala is also known as the fear center of the brain. This is where the "flight or fight" response originates. It helps to alert the other part of the brain when it senses danger. In turn, it starts the release of specific hormones and the firing of other brain receptors that make the body respond to a threatened danger.

This is a useful process when you are faced with a real threat and a "need for survival" situation. But it can be injurious when it develops into an illogical fear, i.e., fear of being rejected, or fear of speaking in front of people.

Tapping is effective in turning off the amygdala, inter-rupting the stress response, and giving the brain synapses a chance to rewire for a better emotional response to a situation.

Tapping utilizes the mind-body connection by recognizing and incorporating the concepts that disease, pain, and mental wellbeing are in a complex way connected to your emotional states. Tapping your body can help you create a balance in your energy system.

Your body is fully equipped with an energy system traveling along pathways referred to as meridians. When you tap on the endpoints of these meridians, it helps stimulate the energy system. When the origin of the distress is mentally and verbally addressed, areas with blocked energy will be released and allow a natural flow.

As I have earlier mentioned, Tapping is similar to acupuncture. Healing through acupuncture is achieved through the stimulation of the body's meridian and energy flow, just like how Tapping works. The main difference is that acupuncture makes use of needles, and Tapping doesn't require that. So we can say that one advantage Tapping has against acupuncture is the ditching of needles.

The process of Tapping is a painless and simple one. Anyone can learn it, and you can do it to yourself. Tapping can be used with a particular emotional intention towards your experiences and life challenges. With Tapping, you have access to healing, and you have the power to heal yourself by taking control of your life and destiny.

When Tapping on a basic level, you will need to focus on any negative emotions you are experiencing. This may be an unresolved problem, fear, bad memory, worry, or just anything that bothers you. As you sustain your mental focus on what's at hand, use your fingertips to tap on the specific meridian points of the body, about 5–7 times. There are 12 major meridian points that mirror each side of our body and connect to an internal organ, although the EFT focuses mainly on nine. I will highlight the nine points and where they are located.

- Head (The governing vessel): center, crown, and top of your head. (four fingers)
- Karate chop (The small intestine meridian): below the fingers, the outer hand. (four fingers)
- Under the eye (Stomach Meridian): hard spot under the eye that connects with the cheekbone. (two fingers)
- Eyebrow (Bladder meridian): close to the nose bridge, the inner edges of the eyebrow (two fingers)
- Chin (Central vessel): between the chin and bottom lower lip
- Side of eye (Gallbladder meridian): the hard spot in between the temple and eye. (two fingers)
- Under the arm (Spleen Meridian): four inches below the armpit on your side (four fingers)
- Beginning of collarbone (Kidney Meridian): below the hard ridge of the collarbone (four fingers)

- Under the nose (Governing vessel): the point between the upper lip and bottom of the nose (two fingers)

When you concentrate on negative emotions and tap on these meridian points, your body's energy system and the brain's limbic system engage and thereby encourage a sense of safety. Based on the proof the scientific field of epigenetics gave, there will be external changes (your physical and mental health) when you change your internal environment (beliefs and emotions).

WHAT DOES RESEARCH SAY ABOUT TAPPING?

Just like with most healing art that utilizes ancient wisdom in their practice, Tapping also has its critics. In fact, some psychologists and doctors are quick to dismiss the proof of its healing effect despite ample evidence from case studies, practitioner reports, clinical traits, and testimonies from those who have used Tapping.

Over the years, Tapping has gained popularity, and there has been a growing number of research studies proving that Tapping gives real and lasting healing. Research has suggested that Tapping takes away conditions that medications, hospital treatments, and therapy have failed to resolve.

All around the world, different studies have continued to assert the claim on Tapping, and I have compiled some of them so that you can see for yourself. In this section, we will be looking at some scientific evidence that has supported the healing power of EFT for anxiety and depression.

According to a 2019 study that involved 203 participants, there was a test carried out to see the psychological symptoms and physical reactions of individuals that were attending the EFT workshops. The majority of people in this study were women over the age of 50 (Bach et al., 2019).

After the workshop, the researchers reported that there was a great reduction in the participant's anxiety and depression symptoms, as well as in their cravings and level of pain. There was also an improvement in their level of happiness.

Research has also suggested that physical measures can improve blood pressure, heart rate, and the level of stress hormone. According to a 2016 review of fourteen studies on EFT, people who made use of EFT experienced a great reduction in anxiety. The author does recommend that more studies should be carried out to compare standard treatments like cognitive behavioral theory (CBT) with EFT. (Clond, 2016)

Also in 2016, a random and controlled trial carried out a comparison of how effective CBT and EFT is in the treatment of people with anxiety. The study comprised ten people who enrolled in an 8-week program or either EFT or CBT. The results of this trial showed that both CBT and EFT worked as they reduced the symptoms of anxiety.

Another research that involved students with anxiety revealed that EFT was able to help them feel more relaxed and calm.

Not only these studies I have highlighted, but several others have suggested that EFT is effective when treating a condition like anxiety.

Some of these studies are small and limited, and the criticism is that some of the older studies may have flaws in their methods, suggesting that the results are defective and shouldn't be relied on. While more research is needed before definitive conclusions can be drawn on the effectiveness of EFT, the fact remains that it is an option to consider when you want to feel relief.

EFT TAPPING SEQUENCE

As earlier mentioned, Tapping can be used to resolve different health issues. It is important to know how to use it. This brings us to the EFT Tapping sequence, how it works, and how to do it.

So basically, this is how a basic Tapping sequence works:

Identify the problem.

First, for this technique to be effective, you need to identify the problem you want to focus on. What is your fear? This can be general anxiety or a particular issue or situation that makes you feel anxious. This will be your main point as you start Tapping. Focus on that particular fear—this will help to enhance your result.

Take into consideration the situation or problem.

After identifying the problem, the next thing to do is to consider the situation. How exactly do you feel? Then set a yardstick for the level of the situation's intensity. Using a scale of 0 to 10, rate the intensity level of your anxiety. The 10 represents the highest level, while the zero represents the lowest level. Establishing the yardstick will help you observe your progress after you complete an EFT sequence. At the end of the sequence, if your intensity level was 5 compared to the 10 that you started with, then you have recorded a 50% improvement level.

Create a setup declaration.

Before Tapping, you need to have a phrase or statement that describes what you are addressing. The declaration comes with two goals—to acknowledge the issues you are trying to deal with, and a clear assertion of yourself irrespective of the issue.

Your setup statements can be:

- *"Although I am feeling this anxiety, I still accept myself passionately and totally."*
- *"Although I am having trouble breathing, I still accept myself passionately and totally."*
- *"Although I am feeling anxious about my upcoming interview, I still accept myself passionately and totally."*
- *"Although I am feeling anxious about being broke and trapped in a financial situation, I still accept myself passionately and totally."*
- *"Although I am still panicking about how things will turn out, I still accept myself passionately and totally."*
- *"Although I am worried about how I am going to approach my boss and ask for a raise, I still accept myself passionately and totally."*

The setup statements are not limited to the above; you can alter the examples so that they can fit your situation. Whichever you use, just make sure it addresses your problem and not that of someone else. For example, it is wrong to say,

"Although my friend is troubled, I still accept myself passionately and totally."

Now you can start Tapping!

- With your four fingers on one of your hands, start Tapping the Karate Chop (KC) point of your other hand. Remember that the Karate Chop Point is the opposite side of the thumb, the outer part of the hand (edge).
- Now, put your setup declaration to use by repeating it aloud three times, as you simultaneously tap the Karate Chop point.
- Take a deep breath.
- Next, tap each of the remaining eight meridian points in the sequence. I will be listing them below. Tap each of the points for about 5–7 times.

Eyebrow Point (EB)
Side of Eye (SE)
Under Eye (UE)
Under Nose (UN)
Chin Point (CP)
Collarbone Point (CB)
Under Arm (UA)
Top of Head (TH)

- As you are Tapping on the meridian points, repeat a reminder phrase. For instance, "my brokenness" or "my worry" or "my anxiety" or "my anxiety." The reminder phrase will mentally help you focus on the problem.
- Pause and take another deep breath.
- You have now completed this sequence.
- After completing the sequence, you need to focus on the issue again. When compared to a few minutes ago, is your anxiety level intense? Use a scale of 0 to 10 to give it a rating. Is there a shift in the rating? If the level of your anxiety is higher than 3, then you need to take another round of Tapping. You need to keep Tapping through the sequence until you notice that your symptom is gone or, at least, greatly reduced.

In the next sequence, you can slightly change your setup declarations to take a record of the fact that you are putting in an effort to fix the issue or your zeal to see progress. For instance, you can slightly change it to:

- "Although I still have some anxiety, I accept myself passionately and totally."
- "Although I am still facing financial challenges, I accept myself passionately and totally."

- "Although I am still worried about how to approach my boss for a raise, I still accept myself passionately and totally." And the list goes on and on.

What you have just done is focus on dismissing your current anxiety. Now you can work on bringing some positive energy to take the place of the anxiety. The approach you are using is unlike the traditional "positive thinking." With this approach, you are not trying to hide the anxiety and stress you are feeling with a façade of untrue affirmations or trying to be dishonest with yourself. What you are doing is dealing and confronting the anxiety, together with the related negative emotions, and offering yourself a passionate and total acceptance to yourself and your feelings.

After clearing up your emotional dirt, you can now turn your vibrations and thoughts to the positive.

Tapping isn't just a mental trick; it is so much more. And this is why it is more effective than the other positive thinking techniques you may have tried. By Tapping, you are changing your body's energy and biochemistry to a more positive course.

Here are some positive phrases you can make use of:

- *"I am hopeful in my ability to change."*
- *"I am in love with the person I am."*

- *"I am happy with the positive changes I see."*
- *"I am becoming a more cheerful and relaxed person."*
- *"I am achieving a lot."*
- *"I am enjoying the peace and calmness I have."*

The positive phrases above can be used with the same sequence of the Tapping points I have given you.

Now that you know how to Tap, let me give you some tips to guide you through the Tapping sequence and make sure you are using the technique correctly. What's the use of all that you have read in this section if Tapping isn't done in the right way?

So, below are the tips:

- When Tapping, use firm but moderate pressure. It should be the same as testing a melon to see if it is ripe or using your hands to drum on top of a table.
- When Tapping, make use of all four of your fingers, or the first two fingers—the index finger and the middle finger. The two fingers are mostly used for sensitive areas like around your eyes, while the four fingers are used in wide areas.
- Don't use your fingernails to Tap; use your fingertips.

- You can Tap both sides of your body or just one side. The eight meridian points are balanced on either side of your body.

Conclusively, EFT Tapping has so far proven to be an alternative treatment for some physical and health conditions. At the very least, Tapping will help you focus your attention on important things and reduce your disturbing thoughts. As mentioned earlier, research supports it and has indicated that it is an effective treatment for anxiety. Although many people have found EFT helpful, it isn't advisable to rely upon it in isolation. If you are considering using EFT, you should speak to your doctor first.

While it is possible that self-treatment with Tapping can make some people feel better and reduce their symptoms, it is also important that you seek professional help when you experience emotional and physical issues.

In the next chapter, we'll be looking at another great technique that is effective in treating anxiety. This technique is also easy to do and does not require help from someone else. Stay with me as we explore mindfulness and how to do it in the next chapter.

8

MINDFULNESS: HOW TO DO IT AND
HOW IT CAN HELP YOU

Mindfulness is the ability to be fully conscious of the present and aware of what you are doing and where you are, and not overwhelmed or reactive by what's going on around you. We are naturally mindful as humans; all we have to do is practice it daily, and it will become habitual.

Each time you bring awareness to your state of mind through your emotions and thoughts, or to what you're directly experiencing through your senses, you're mindful. Current research shows that when you groom your brain to be mindful, you're reshaping your brain's physical structure to help reduce anxiety.

Each time you practice meditation, you venture into the workings of your mind: your sensations (the cool breeze blowing on your skin), your emotions (hate that, love this, loathe that, crave this) and even your thoughts (you may imagine how weird it would be to see an elephant playing the trumpet).

Practicing mindfulness aids you to focus your attention on the present. It draws your focus away from worries about the past or the future. Thus, it is a great tool for managing anxiety. It has several physical and psychological benefits and can be practiced easily at home. Try to practice 3–4 times a week to incorporate mindfulness into your life and help you to manage anxiety symptoms.

It enables you to suspend judgment and unleash your curiosity about your mind's activities and approach your experience with kindness and warmth toward yourself and others.

It helps to teach us how to respond to stress with awareness rather than acting on instinct.

It encourages us to accept our emotions, making it easy to identify and process them, and it enables you to see things from different points of view.

SEVERAL BENEFITS:

Many medical practitioners have done in-depth investigations on the benefits of mindfulness. The overall evidence shows that meditation helps improve various conditions such as anxiety, stress, depression, pain, high blood pressure, and insomnia. Preliminary research also shows that meditation helps people with fibromyalgia and asthma. Meditation also has been shown to improve attention, sleep, and diabetes control, and decrease job burnout. In summary, meditation helps you experience emotions and thoughts with greater acceptance and balance.

Mindfulness improves wellbeing.

Improving the level of mindfulness supports many attitudes that lead to a more satisfying life. Mindfulness makes it easier to manage the pleasures in life as they occur, helps you become fully engaged in activities, and improves your ability to deal with stressful events. Being mindful reduces your chances of getting caught up in worries about regrets over the past, or a future event you think may go wrong. A mindful person is less preoccupied with concerns about self-esteem and success, and can easily form deep connections with others.

· · ·

Mindfulness improves physical health.

Apart from giving you greater wellbeing, scientists have discovered that mindfulness helps improve our physical health in several ways. Mindfulness techniques can treat heart disease, help relieve stress, lower blood pressure, improve sleep, reduce chronic pain, and alleviate gastrointestinal difficulties.

Mindfulness improves mental health.

In recent investigations by psychotherapists, mindfulness meditation is great for treating several problems such as anxiety disorders, depression, eating disorders, substance abuse, and couple's conflict.

Body awareness.

This has to do with noticing sensations in the body. Current findings by those who have used mindfulness techniques show that it increases perceptions of body awareness.

Focused attention.

Mindfulness increases the ability to focus attention. Neuroimaging studies show that mindfulness improves the activation of the brain area known as the anterior cingulate cortex (ACC). This area is involved in attention and executive function, and enables us to focus attention on the present rather than being distracted by worry.

Self-perception.

Research found that two months of mindfulness practice changes self-perspective and increases self-esteem and self-acceptance.

Physical health.

Besides reducing anxiety, mindfulness has other health benefits such as reduced cortisol levels and blood pressure.

MINDFULNESS TECHNIQUES

Mindfulness can be practiced in several ways, but each mindfulness technique aims to achieve total control over feelings and emotions by engaging in focused relaxation and deliberately paying attention to sensations and thoughts without judgment. This practice allows the mind to refocus on the present. All mindfulness techniques are a form of meditation.

Basic mindfulness meditation: This has to do with sitting quietly and focusing on breathing or on a word (mantra) that you repeat silently. Let your thoughts flow without any judgment, and ensure you return your focus to your mantra or breath.

Body sensations: In this mindfulness technique, when you notice subtle sensations in the body such as tingling or itching, let them pass without judgment. You have to notice each part of your body in sequence from head to toe.

Sensory: Notice sounds, sights, smells, touches, and tastes. You have to name them accordingly "sound," "sight," "smell," "touch," or "taste," without judgment and let them pass.

Emotions: You have to permit emotions to be present without judgment. You need to practice a relaxed and steady naming of emotions: "anger," "frustration," "joy." Accept the presence of each emotion without judgment and let them pass.

Urge surfing: With this mindfulness technique, you have to cope with cravings (for addictive behaviors or substances) and let them pass. Also, you have to notice how your body feels when the craving comes. Finally, you have to replace the wish for the craving with the knowledge that it will subside.

All these techniques build concentration practices by following the same key principles:

Go with the flow.

To begin mindfulness meditation, you have to establish concentration by observing the flow of inner emotions, thoughts, and bodily sensations without judging them as bad or good.

Pay attention.

The external sensations such as sounds, sights, and touch that you notice during meditation make up your moment-to-moment experience. The problem is not to latch onto a particular sensation, idea, emotion, or to get caught in thinking about the future or past. Instead, you have to watch what comes and goes in your mind and realize the mental habits that give you a feeling of suffering or wellbeing.

Stay with it.

From the onset, this process may not seem relaxing at all, but over time it gives you greater self-awareness and happiness as you become comfortable with a wider and wider range of your experiences.

MINDFULNESS TRICKS TO MANAGE ANXIETY

Apply these mindfulness tricks to ease anxiety and ease your mind.

Create a worry diary: It is difficult to rationally analyze worrisome thoughts as they swirl and dance through your innocent mind. By writing them on a paper, they will be easier to tackle using a structured set of questions. When this is done accurately with a worry diary, you can find the truth, which will help you stop worrying about what is likely to occur.

Step 1: Write down your worries: When your worries start interfering with daily activities or when you start feeling overwhelmed, take some minutes to write down exactly what you are worrying about.

Why you need to write down your worries:

1. Writing them down eliminates some of their effect over you. You no longer have to meditate over them once you have them in your notebook.
2. Discharging your worries to the notebook frees up some headspace and helps you think clearly.
3. Once you have all your worries written down, you can commence a structured worry-challenging exercise.

Step 2: Clarify Your Worries: After writing down all your worries, you need to clarify and identify them in writing. Afterward, you can start evaluating and challenging these distressing thoughts.

To clarify your worries, you need to ask yourself the following questions.

- What bad thing do I think is going to take place?
- What is the chance that this bad thing is going to happen?
- What are my emotions at the moment?
- What's the force of these emotions?

For instance:

- I am worried the transaction into my account won't be completed.
- I think something is wrong with the transaction. I have not gotten any updates from the bank.
- I am feeling anxious right now.
- 75 out of 100

Step 3: Challenge anxious thoughts: In this step, you have to examine how valid your worries are, through challenging questions aimed to elicit truth and reality.

To challenge your worries, ask, and answer the following questions.

- What evidence supports my worry?
- Is there any evidence against my worry?
- In reality, what is the probability that what I am worried about is actually going to happen?
- What's the worst-case scenario?

- What's the best-case scenario?
- What will probably happen?
- Is being fearful about it helping at all?
- Can I cope if my worst-case scenario happens?
- What can I do to remedy the situation?
- Can I see this situation from another dimension?

Step 4: Reframe the situation: After successfully asking and answering the challenge questions, you have to finalize the processing of this worry.

Set an intention: Irrespective of when you do it, setting an intention helps you focus and reminds you why you are doing something. That's why most yoga teachers instruct that you set an intention for your practice each day. If something gives you anxiety—like writing an exam in school—set an intention for it.

For instance, you can set an intention to treat your body with kindness before eating or to care for your body before heading to the gym.

Do a guided mindfulness or meditation practice:
There are many apps and online programs available to enable you to practice a guided meditation without committing to an expensive class or taking up much time.

Doodle or color: Dedicate a couple of minutes to doodle. Invest in a coloring book. This will help eliminate the thoughts that bring you anxiety as your mind gets focused on the coloring book.

Go for a walk: Being outside is a great way to reduce anxiety. Go for a walk, pay attention to the feel of the wind against your skin, the sounds around you, and the smells around you. Ensure your phone doesn't distract you (keep it in your pocket or better yet, at home), and try to stay in the moment by focusing on your environment and your senses.

Wish other people happiness: A few seconds is enough for you to execute this wonderful trick from the author and former Google pioneer Chade-Meng Tan. You have to randomly wish for someone to be happy throughout the day. This practice is all in your head. Try it on your commute, at the gym, at the office, or while you wait in line. If you find yourself annoyed with someone, you have to stop and (mentally) wish them happiness instead.

Look up: Whether you are coming home late or taking out the trash, pause and take a few deep breaths into your stomach as you look up at the stars. With eyes up, let the cosmos remind you that life is bigger than the situation.

Focus on one thing at a time: Your to-do list can be a form of mindfulness if you develop it well and keep to it. Set a timer for five minutes or less and dedicate your full and undivided attention. Don't check your phone, no browsing online, no clicking on notifications. In fact, absolutely no multitasking. Focus on that one task at hand until the timer goes off.

Leave your phone behind: The fact is, you really don't have to take your phone along when going to the next room, when you sit down to eat, or when you go to the bathroom. Keep your phone in the other room, and it will still be there when you are done. Don't worry about it. Sit and breathe before you start eating. You need to create a moment for yourself and your needs in the bathroom or any other place you need to be.

Turn household tasks into a mental break: Relax into the moment instead of obsessing yourself over your to-do list or clutter. Focus on the way the soap flows down the tiles while you clean the bathroom or dance while you do the dishes. Daydream while you fold the laundry. Take a series of slow breaths while you wait for the microwave to stop.

Journal: There is no best or worst way to journal. You can start with a structured five-minute journal, or you could opt for scribbling your thoughts on a random piece of paper. The act of writing can help console the mind and quiet swirling thoughts. Jot down three amazing things that happened today.

Pause at stoplights: Don't time travel or wish to make cars move out of your way when you're running late. Instead, bring your focus inward at every stoplight. While you wait for the stoplights, sit still and upright and take five slow, deep breaths. This exercise may sound easy and meaningless on a leisurely drive, but the benefits will help you when your stress and anxiety level is high.

Log out of all of your social media accounts: It's true that social media has its uses, but it can also interrupt your productivity and contribute to your anxiety. You'll be amazed at how often you check your accounts without thinking. So, log out.

When you actually want to check-in, set an intention, or better still, a time limit. That way, you won't end up feeling guilty for spending 20 minutes looking at a stranger's pet or getting behind on your work.

You may also, if possible, delete some social media accounts. A recent study found that using numerous social media platforms increases the level of anxiety in young adults.

Check out: Steadily trying to be mindful at all times can actually add to stress and anxiety. Know when you need to let your mind wander where it wants to go.

Practicing mindfulness meditation 3–4 times a week can help you bring mindfulness into your life and manage your anxiety. The more you do it, the more effective it gets. Mindfulness works well when coupled with relaxation techniques. In the next chapter, we will explore relaxation techniques so you can combine them for the best outcomes.

EFFECTIVE RELAXATION TECHNIQUES FOR ALL TYPES OF ANXIETY

The whole concept of anxiety means you are tensed and riled up. If you can find a means of relaxing your body when you are anxious, and when you are not, you will reduce the anxiety episodes you suffer, and the severity too. To be relaxed, you have to know how to activate your body's relaxation response. If you master it, it can help you to manage your anxiety.

Several techniques are available that you can use to activate your body's relaxation response. Techniques like deep breathing and progressive muscle relaxation can give you tools you can use anywhere to help manage anxiety as it arises. But even when it hasn't occurred, it will be helpful to you if you can build relaxation into your everyday life to ensure that your anxiety is continually being addressed even before they arise.

When we talk about relaxation, we are not saying you should zone out in front of the TV. While that type of relaxation is great, it does not address the effects of stress and anxiety.

The relaxation technique I speak of is capable of activating your body's natural relaxation response—a state of deep rest that slows breathing and heart rate, lowers blood pressure, and rebalances mind and body.

While people often achieve this state through meditation, there are other relaxation techniques you can employ to achieve it. Try different techniques and activities to see what works best for you, your anxiety, and your lifestyle. A technique that works for your neighbor might not work for you. But since there are several techniques to choose from, there will always be something for you.

DEEP BREATHING:

If you have been anxious before, then you know how fast your breathing becomes. This fast breathing is the body's way of trying to provide the brain with all the nutrients and oxygen it needs to cope with the numerous activities going on in there. But often, the body is unable to meet up, and you will start experiencing symptoms such as breathlessness, lightheadedness, dizziness, and tingly feelings in your hands and feet. Since the heart is beating fast, it also increases blood pressure. These symptoms are frightening, so they lead to further anxiety and panic.

But when you reduce the activity in the brain and effectively reduce the pace of your breathing, these symptoms will reduce or disappear totally, and you can calm yourself down. That is what deep breathing does for you.

It simply involves breathing deeply from your diaphragm. This technique is easy to learn and can be practiced anywhere, which means you can use it to help in the face of an anxiety attack. You can also incorporate it into your everyday living even when you are not having an attack.

It stimulates the vagus nerve, activation relaxation response. The vagus nerve extends from the head, through the neck and chest all the way to the colon. As you stimulate it, it activates your relaxation response, and that action lowers stress levels, reduces your heart rate and blood pressure. It is a cornerstone of many other relaxation practices. Most other relaxation techniques will require that you calm yourself first with deep breathing before starting them. Thus, it can be combined with other relaxing things like baths, aromatherapy, and music.

* * *

Steps for Practicing Deep Breathing:

1. Sit or lie in a comfortable position that will allow you to straighten your back. Place one hand on your stomach and the other on your chest.

2. With your hands in place, inhale in such a manner that the hand on your stomach rises while the other hand remains steady or rises just slightly.

3. Breathe out through your mouth and push out all inhaled air. Contract your abdominal muscle, ensuring that only the hand on your stomach moves, while the hand on your chest stays steady.

4. Continue the process, each time ensuring that your stomach lowers and rises as much as it can. Both breathing should be done slowly for the best impact.

If you discover that you can breathe better from your stomach when lying down than when sitting, then always lay down when practicing your deep breathing. With your back on the ground, you can place a small book on your stomach and ensure that the book rises when you breathe in and falls when you breathe out.

The steps above are straightforward enough, but if you are having issues with following it, you can get videos and apps that will guide you through. The procedure is mostly similar.

PROGRESSIVE MUSCLE RELAXATION

Most times, when you are anxious or stressed, your body reacts with muscle tension. This exercise helps you relieve that tension. The idea here is that if you know how to do it even when you are not tense, you can just do it easily and relieve your body of the tension it will be subjected to when you are anxious.

It is a two-step process that involves systematically tensing and relaxing different muscle groups in your body. PMR (Progressive Muscle Relaxation) helps you familiarize yourself with what tension and relaxation feel like in different parts of your body. But you can only gain such intimate familiarity with regular practice. That intimate familiarity will help you promptly detect and react to the first signs of muscular tension. It is this muscular tension that accompanies stress that eventually puts you in a state of tension. So when you cut out the muscular tension, you can relax your body, and your mind will be relaxed as well. That is because as the body relaxes, so does the mind.

Progressive muscle relaxation can give you additional stress relief when you combine it with deep breathing.

* * *

Steps for Practicing Progressive Muscle Relaxation

Before you start this exercise, ensure that you do not have any condition that can be aggravated by this exercise, such as muscle spasms, back pains, or any underlying serious injuries. You can consult with your physician if you are not sure.

Seeing how the exercise is all about tensing and relaxing certain muscles, it is advisable you start from your feet and proceed to your face, taking care that no muscle is left out.

Proceed in the following manner:

1. Get comfortable by loosening any tight outfit and being bare-footed.
2. Practice deep breathing for a few minutes, ensuring that you breathe deeply and slowly.
3. When you are ready, start with your right leg. Inhale and tense the muscle group, hold for ten seconds.
4. Breathe out and relax the muscle group suddenly and completely. Take note of the word "suddenly." Don't make the mistake of relaxing it gradually. As you slowly relax the muscle, take note of how tension flows away from your leg and how limp and loose it feels afterward.

5. Let your body relax for 10–20 seconds, then work on your next muscle group, in this case, your left leg. Follow the same sequence of tensing and releasing your muscles described above.

6. From your left leg, work the other relevant muscles as follows:

- For your buttocks, press them together tightly.
- For your stomach, tense by sucking it into a tight knot and releasing it gradually.
- For the chest, inhale deeply and hold for about ten seconds.
- For your hands, clench them for tension and slow-release tension by opening them.
- For your wrists and forearms, extend them and push your hands back at your wrist.
- For your biceps and upper arms, clench your hands first, then bend your arms at your elbow and flex the biceps.
- For your shoulders, shrug them by raising them towards your ears.
- For the back of the neck, press it against the floor or chair.
- For your cheeks and jaws, smile as widely as possible.

- For the muscles around your mouth, tense them by pressing your lips together tightly.
- For your eyes, close them as tightly as possible. Note that this exercise cannot be done while wearing contact lenses. Remove them first, and after the exercise, you can put them back in.
- For your forehead, wrinkle it into a deep frown.

If you are new to progressive muscle relaxation, it might be helpful for you to use video or audio resources so that you will get conversant with the muscle groups and how to transition between them. You can check your local library, or use online video resources for this purpose.

BODY SCAN MEDITATION

The idea here is that when we are stressed, most of the physical discomfort we feel, such as tense muscles, pains, and headaches are mostly connected with our emotional state. Therefore, when you perform the body scan meditation, you are aiming to release the tension that you might not have noticed that you are experiencing.

In this technique, you will focus attention on various parts of your body so you can detect any bodily sensation that you may be having. It is advisable to start with your feet and work up, focusing on how each part of the body feels. As you do this, do not label any feeling as good or bad. Just be aware of them so you can learn from them so you can better manage them.

This relaxation technique breaks the cycle of physical and psychological tension that we often have as humans.

Here is how you can practice it:

1. Start by getting cozy and by getting into a comfortable position where you can easily stretch your limbs.
2. Close your eyes so you can truly focus on your body parts. Start by focusing on your breath, and notice the sensation of how your breath fills and leaves your lungs as you breathe.
3. It is advised you start from your leg, but you can start from any area of your body, just ensure you don't leave out any body part.
4. Any spot you choose to start, focus on that portion as you breathe slowly and deeply. Try to notice any sensation of pain, discomfort, tension, or anything unusual. Don't rush it; ensure you observe the sensation, if any. Slowly release your mental awareness on this body part before proceeding to other parts.

5. As you proceed, do not allow your thoughts to drift off. Remain in the moment.

When you finish, lie still for a while and notice how your entire body feels. Throughout the exercise, ensure that you give yourself all the time you need to truly investigate and experience every part of your body.

VISUALIZATION

This relaxation technique involves imagining a scene in which you feel peaceful and free. You are to choose any setting that is most calming to you. It may be a movie scene, a favorite childhood spot, a sunny beach, or whatever scene that calms you. Try to let go of all tension and anxiety in the scene. It is also known as guided imagery. You can practice it on your own or with an app, listening aid, or video resource.

You can practice visualization through the following steps:

- Start by getting into a comfortable position in a comfortable and quiet place.
- Close your eyes and imagine your desired place.
- As you picture and imagine the place, be as detailed as possible. You can do that by engaging all your senses which are sight, smell, taste, sound, and feel. For instance, if your peaceful spot is a tropical

beach, try to see the waves, hear birds chirping in the distance and the waves crashing, and feel the water against your feet, and so on.

- Try to enjoy what you are feeling while letting yourself forget all the worries, tension, and anxiety you may be having.

When you feel like you have relieved yourself of every tension, you may gently open your eyes and return back to the present.

SELF-MASSAGE

You must have heard of people going to spas and health clubs to get a massage from professionals at exorbitant prices. That's because it can be massaging yourself or receiving a massage from someone else that reduces stress, relieves pain, and eases muscle tension. If you can get someone to massage you, you should, but if you can't, take a few minutes to self-massage between daily tasks or the end of the day. You can enhance the relaxation you get by combining it with mindfulness, deep breathing, or aromatherapy. You can also use scented lotions and aromatic oil to enhance relaxation.

You can carry out self-massage through the following steps:

1. Knead the muscles of your shoulder and the back of your neck. To do this, make a loose fist with your hands and drum quickly on the back of your neck. Next, massage the base of your skull by making tiny circles there with your fingers. Then tap your scalp with your fingers moving from side to side.

2. Massage your face by making a tiny circle with your fingertips. Take note that you massage your temples, forehead, and jaw muscles properly.

RHYTHMIC MOVEMENTS/MINDFUL EXERCISE

A rhythmic exercise that gets you in a flow of regular movement can produce a relaxation response. Examples of such rhythmic movements are running, swimming, walking, dancing, rowing, and climbing. You can combine this with mindfulness by paying attention to how your body feels in the moment rather than focusing on your anxiety.

If in the process of practicing this technique, your mind wanders to other thoughts, try and refocus yourself by gently returning your thought to the sensations in your body parts.

YOGA/TAI CHI

Tai chi and yoga have physical benefits as well as relaxation benefits for managing anxiety. If you are new to yoga and tai chi, it is best to start with a class because injuries can occur if it is performed wrong. Once you have learned the basics, then you can start practicing alone and modifying it to suit your personality and needs.

Yoga is a sequence of stationary and moving poses, combined with deep breathing to relieve stress and anxiety. It can also be used to improve one's stamina, balance, flexibility, and strength. The types of yoga that focus on slow, steady movement, deep breathing, and gentle stretching are best for anxiety management. Examples are Satyananda, Power and Hatha.

Tai chi is slow, flowing body movements that force you to focus on the movement and your breathing, thereby clearing your mind. It is believed that by focusing on these flows, you can remain in the present, and that is what clears your mind and brings you relaxation.

Tai chi is best learned in a class. If you feel this is a relaxation technique that you want to explore, consider signing up with a fitness class in your neighborhood that offers tai chi classes. As with yoga, once you have learned the basics, you can start practicing alone and tailoring your practice as you desire.

OTHER FORMS OF RELAXATION

Deliberate relaxation can also come in the form of doing activities you enjoy and focusing on those activities (mindfulness) rather than your anxiety. This might include

- Art - drawing/painting/coloring/crafting
- Reading
- Long bath listening to soothing music
- Listening to music

None of the relaxation techniques we've discussed here will yield benefits straightaway. It takes time and practice before you will start reaping any meaningful benefits. Try not to skip days, but even if you do, don't allow it to stop you. Start again and keep going with the goal in your mind.

It is best if you can set up a time in your daily schedule when you will practice any of these relaxation techniques so that when that time is approaching, your body will start entering the mood.

In conclusion, relaxation techniques can be helpful for relieving moderate anxiety. But when it is extreme, you may need to consult a doctor and get professional treatment. In the next chapter, we will discuss some of the therapy and medication options available to you if these relaxation techniques we've discussed don't work for you.

THERAPY AND MEDICATION: WHAT ARE YOUR OPTIONS?

Most people can manage their anxiety through self-help strategies and lifestyle changes, but sometimes, your symptoms may be so great that you require professional help. If self-help methods aren't working for you, you just might need something a little extra, but be sure you gave self-help strategies a fair chance.

The most used types of therapy for anxiety disorders are cognitive behavioral therapy (CBT) and exposure therapy (ET). If these ones fail, medication can be prescribed, but this varies between patients, and your therapist will devise the right treatment plan for you depending on your type of disorder and the severity.

In this chapter, we will explore the therapy and medication options that are available to you.

I know you badly want to practice the self-help strategies that we discussed in the previous chapter. But if you have tried and your symptoms prove to be too big for them, you have to do the right thing. The general guide is that once your symptoms (worries, fears, or anxiety) are so significant that they have started bringing distress to you and disrupting your daily routine. You have to involve a professional who will either follow you up with therapy or medication. While you are on therapy and medication, you can continue with the self-help strategies as they can still help you manage your anxiety, but don't substitute them for professional help when there is a need for one.

If you are experiencing a lot of physical symptoms, start with a medical checkup. That is because sometimes anxiety can be caused by a medical condition such as asthma, hypoglycemia, and thyroid problems. Therefore, a checkup rules out the possibility that your symptoms are due to one of these medical conditions. Once it has been proven with a checkup that you do not have any medical condition that can manifest itself in the form of the symptoms you are getting, then you may have one of the anxiety disorders.

Once medical problems have been ruled out, consult a therapist who specializes in anxiety disorders. They will conduct some assessments to be sure that what you have is anxiety, and they will tell which of the anxiety disorders you have and the probable cause. Since it is possible for certain medications to cause you anxiety, the mental expert will also go over all your prescriptions to be sure you are not on any risky medications. Prescriptions, such as over-the-counter medications and recreational drugs, will be checked. Then they will devise a treatment plan tailored to your needs.

MEDICATIONS

Medication is sometimes prescribed for anxiety disorders, but it is usually only a temporary measure to relieve symptoms. It is particularly essential when your anxiety is enough to stop you from functioning. However, medications must be prescribed and closely monitored by a mental health expert because anxiety medications can be addictive and cause undesirable side effects.

This is why it should be your last line of defense. You should only use it when every other thing we've discussed fails. You should try changes in lifestyle, therapy, exercise, and the self-help strategies we discussed. Oftentimes, they will be all you need. If, however, they fail, you can consider medication.

Medication for GAD

With GAD, medications are temporary measures to help relieve you of your symptoms at the beginning of your treatment. For long-term treatment, therapy will be mostly used as they have more long-term success than medications.

A medication commonly prescribed for GAD includes:

- Buspirone: It is an anti-anxiety drug that is generally considered as the safest medication for GAD. It only serves to reduce anxiety symptoms and not to eliminate the anxiety. It can be identified by the brand name "Buspar."
- Benzodiazepines: This is another anti-anxiety drug like buspirone, but it acts faster. It can act anywhere between half an hour to an hour. The problem with it is that users can become physically and psychologically dependent on it when they use it for a few weeks. Hence, you should only use this medication if your symptoms are severe and paralyzing, and nothing else is working for you.
- Antidepressants: Antidepressants can provide you with relief from anxiety, but it doesn't come immediately. You won't feel the full effect until you use it for up to six weeks and above. For some people, antidepressants may not be suitable because it may cause them to have sleep problems, nausea, or other mild side effects. If you notice that you are reacting to any antidepressants prescribed by your qualified mental health expert, inform them

immediately so they can place you on a different product line.

Medication for SAD

The medications that are used for SAD are mostly used as a means to silence symptoms and not cure them altogether. This is the reason it is mostly used with therapy and other self-care practices we've discussed. The belief is that while the medication relieves symptoms, the therapy and self-care processes can help you look for a permanent cure because those ones can address the main cause of the anxiety, not just tackling the symptoms.

A medication commonly prescribed for SAD includes:

- Beta-blockers: This medication relieves performance anxiety. They are used to control the physical symptoms of social anxiety such as shortness of breath, shaky hands or voice, rapid heartbeat, and sweating. However, they cannot affect the emotional symptoms of anxiety. It is typically prescribed for patients with heart disease. A common example of beta-blockers is propranolol (Inderal). To use it, you will have to take it an hour before you encounter a social anxiety trigger such as public speaking. Studies show that it works, as it

helps patients perform in the midst of social
phobia.

- Benzodiazepines: This medication can also be used
  for SAD since it is generally an anti-anxiety
  medication. It works by boosting the activity of
  gamma-aminobutyric acid (an inhibitory
  neurotransmitter). In layman terms, it suppresses
  the signal that travels through the neural pathway.
  Once these signals are suppressed, the individual
  experiences a calming of anxiety symptoms. Even
  though they are fast in action, the problem with
  them, as we noted before, is that they are sedative
  and addictive. Hence, they should be used only
  when other methods have failed.

- Antidepressants: The antidepressants we discussed
  above can also be useful for SAD, especially when
  the disorder is very severe.

Medication for OCD

Medication is rarely effective for treating OCD, but sometimes antidepressants are prescribed alongside other therapies. Medications alone cannot relieve the symptoms.
Instead, exposure and response prevention techniques
described earlier in this book are mostly used for treating
OCD. Cognitive therapy is also used. Cognitive therapy

focuses on handling the catastrophic thoughts that cause you the symptoms you feel.

THERAPIES FOR ANXIETY DISORDERS

Therapies are better for anxiety disorders because they uncover the underlying causes of the anxiety you feel. It will help you to learn how to relax and how to look at the situation in a new and less frightening angle. It will also help you develop better coping skills. In summary, therapies equip you with the tools you need to combat anxiety and teach you how to use them.

Anxiety disorders respond well to therapy, and often quickly. The American Psychological Association says that it takes from eight to ten correctly done sessions for people to improve significantly. Therefore, it is mostly a short-term treatment even though it takes longer when compared to medication.

Your therapist will come up with the best plan for you, but two of the most common treatments for anxiety disorders are cognitive behavioral therapy (CBT) and exposure therapy, which focus on the behavior rather than the cause. Most times, the type of anxiety and its severity will determine the treatment approach to be adopted.

These therapies can be conducted for an individual or a group of people—both work.

Cognitive Behavioral Therapy (CBT)

This therapy teaches you some new ways you can start thinking and behaving to reduce or eliminate your anxiety disorder. Fundamentally, it addresses the negative patterns in the way you look at yourself and the world around you. It is these patterns that cause you to have anxiety disorders. It is one of the most effective and widely used treatments for anxiety available. It can be administered by a psychiatrist, psychologist, counselor, or other qualified therapists. It helps you identify and challenge the negative thinking patterns fueling your anxiety.

Several research studies have been done to enquire about the efficacy of CBT as a treatment for anxiety and most of the point to the fact that it is an effective therapy. These studies have discovered that CBT is effective against SAD, GAD, phobias, panic disorders, and many other related illnesses.

From the name "cognitive behavioral therapy," we can see that there are two parts to it, the cognitive part and the behavioral part.

Cognitive therapy is involved with the examination of all the negative thoughts and distortions that you have that cause you anxiety. Behavioral therapy, on the other hand, examines how you behave or react to the objects or situations that trigger your anxiety.

It is our thoughts about an external event that controls our moods, not the external events around us, and that is what CBT is based on. If that is the case, then it is your perception of the situations around you that decides how you feel, not the situations themselves.

Let me demonstrate with this example. If someone invites you for a party with some friends, you may react to it in two broad ways. The first is that you may be happy because parties are fun and you like to meet new people. If you react to the invitation this way, you will be excited and happy. But if you start telling yourself that you don't know how to mingle with people, you don't look presentable enough, and that you will embarrass yourself, the invitation brings you sadness and anxiety.

So you see how different perceptions of an external situation (the invitation) affected your mood in two different ways. It boils down to your attitude and beliefs about situations. If you have anxiety disorders, you will always look at things negatively, and that will fuel your anxiety and fear. CBT, therefore, is targeted at discovering those negative thoughts and correcting them. Once it helps you to change the way you think, you can change the way you feel.

The five components of CBT for anxiety are:

1. Education: As I said earlier, the best point for you to start your fight against any of the anxiety disorders is education. You have to become an expert in that field, and CBT emphasizes that too. CBT teaches that when you understand your anxiety, you will be more accepting and proactive when dealing with it.

2. Monitoring: Once you have educated yourself on your anxiety, the next thing is monitoring the anxiety, discovering your triggers, and noting the intensity of your anxiety with different triggers. With that, you can get a good perspective of your anxiety, and when you start self-care strategies, you can monitor your progress.

3. Physical Control Strategies: Remember how an anxiety disorder gets the better of you by destabilizing you physically, CBT counters that by teaching you relaxation techniques, some of which we discussed in the previous chapter.

4. Cognitive Control Strategies: This aspect of CBT shows you how you can evaluate the thinking pattern that causes you anxiety so that you can begin to alter them. You can alter them by challenging them. As you challenge them, your fears reduce.

5. Behavioral Strategies: CBT teaches you that avoiding the situations you fear is not the best for you; rather, you should summon the courage to tackle them. One way to do that is to imagine the things you fear and put your focus on them. Don't try to escape them. With time, you will become less anxious and gain more control.

The procedure for applying CBT is as follows: identifying a negative thought, challenging the thoughts, and replacing the negative thought with better and realistic thoughts.

For instance, a distortive thought might be: if I climb up that podium to talk to these people, I might pass out. This is you predicting the worst for yourself even when there are other more realistic and better outcomes such as speaking fluently and receiving a standing ovation. You will still tell yourself that if you pass out, it will be a disgrace to you, and people will not take you seriously.

You can replace that negative thought with a more realistic one, such as "I have never passed out on the podium before." You can as well tell yourself that even if you pass out, it will not be so terrible since you will come on soon and you won't be the first person to pass out on a podium.

Your CBT will also help you know when you are beginning to blow things out of proportion so you can return back to more realistic thinking.

Exposure Therapy (ET)

I know how it is much easier to avoid any anxiety-inducing situation because anxiety is not a great thing to feel. So people always try to avoid any situation that can bring them face to face with anxiety. This is why somebody who is scared of flying will prefer to spend several hours on the road to escape their fears. ET helps you to confront your anxieties and fears in a controlled, safe environment. It works on the principle that as you are gradually exposed to your fear (object or situation), either in reality or imagination, your anxiety will start diminishing, and you will gain a greater sense of control over them. That's because as you face the fear and you are not harmed as you thought, you will begin to see how unfounded your fears truly are.

For this therapy, the therapist will ask you to imagine the scary situation, or you may have to confront it. It may be conducted alone or combined with CBT. The therapist will use systematic desensitization when exposing the patient to the anxiety. That will mean starting from small fears and moving to tougher ones. For instance, if you are scared of flying, you may start by looking at photos of planes. After conquering that, you can watch videos of planes in flight, then watch planes as they take off, book a plane ticket, pack for a flight, get on a plane and, eventually, take the flight.

GUIDE FOR APPLICATION OF THERAPIES FOR ANXIETY DISORDERS

As you would expect, some therapies are more effective for some anxiety disorders more than others. Therapies can be used alone or combined with others if need be. Below is a general guide:

- For GAD & SAD, CBT is often used.
- For OCD, a combination of CBT and ERP is often used.
- Sometimes group therapy is recommended, particularly for CBT.

In conclusion, when all the self-help strategies we've discussed have failed, you can fall back to therapy and medication. They can be done differently or combined if there is a need. Whichever one you are going for, ensure that you are doing it with a qualified mental health expert who specializes in anxiety disorders. While the medications will give you faster results, the therapies offer more long-lasting benefits, even though it might take time before you can see notable results.

FINAL WORDS

Anxiety disorders are common mental conditions that are affecting several people daily. It can be challenging for those who have these anxiety disorders. That is because people who suffer from these disorders do not try to understand them. Hence, they are always anxious because they fear what they don't know. But that is not you. You, my friend, have spent time reading this book. My best bet is that you are already beginning to see a glimpse of hope. I want to tell you that if you follow the tips I have shared in this book, you will soon be free from any anxiety disorder that has caged your life.

Now, let's quickly remind ourselves of the talking points so that they can be fresh in your mind as you go all out against that anxiety disorder. We started our discussion by looking at anxiety and the different types of anxiety disorders. I hope you were able to pick the one you have from the lot. We said anxiety, on its own, is normal, but when it starts to interfere with your life and is continuously present, it becomes a disorder. There are seven types of disorder, but three are more common and usually more severe. They include generalized anxiety disorder (GAD), social anxiety disorder (SAD), obsessive-compulsive disorder (OCD), panic disorder, phobias and irrational fears, post-traumatic stress disorder (PTSD), and separation anxiety disorder.

The symptoms of anxiety disorders fall into two broad categories of psychological and physical. They include feelings of dread, expecting the worst, blank mindedness, irritability, difficulty in concentrating for the psychological symptoms and pounding heart, headaches, dizziness, shortness of breath, and so on, for the physical symptoms.

We also took a closer look at anxiety attacks so we can begin to understand why and how they happen. Even though panic attacks and anxiety attacks are somewhat related, they have their differences. Since anxiety attacks can't be medically diagnosed and people living with anxiety often get panic attacks, they are confused for each other. A significant difference between them is that panic attacks are recognized by DSM-5, whereas anxiety attacks are not.

Irrespective of the type of anxiety you may have, certain lifestyle changes can make a significant difference. You have to build your recovery from the disorder on a strong foundation by living a healthy lifestyle. You have to work on your diet because some foods can increase anxiety while some other food can reduce them. You have to add some foods to your diet and also ensure you stick to meal timing. In the same vein, you must eliminate other substances like alcohol and caffeine as they can aggravate symptoms. As you work on your diet, ensure that you often exercise, cut out sources of stress, socialize with people, and get the right amount of sleep.

We also looked at the three major anxiety disorders: GAD, SAD, and OCD. We looked at the symptoms associated with each of them and the coping strategies you can adopt to reduce your symptoms. With most of these anxiety disorders, it is right for you to recognize your triggers and the extent to which they affect you so that you can expect them and act accordingly. While GAD has to do with anxiety and worrying over almost everything, SAD has to do with anxiety when the patient finds themselves in a social setting. OCD is characterized by obsessions and compulsions in which you find yourself doing things even when you know it is illogical. Oftentimes you are doing them because you fear that if you don't, something terrible will happen.

In looking at the self-help strategies you can adopt to fight off anxiety disorders, we looked at emotional freedom technique (EFT), mindfulness, and relaxation technique. EFT is an alternative medicine that is similar to acupuncture. Research shows that it can help you manage stress. Mindfulness enables you to focus your attention on the present so that you can take your mind away from troubling thoughts that cause you anxiety. Relaxation helps you activate the body's relaxation responses so you can better manage anxiety. These self-help techniques have some subdivisions, and we took the time to discuss each one of them. They are mostly things you can do alone except for some that you may need to be taught.

If you've tried self-help strategies and failed, you can try therapy, and if that too fails, you may consider medication. Before going for therapy and medication, check that your symptoms are not due to any underlying medical condition. Once you have ruled that out, have a qualified mental expert take you through therapies and medication. In therapy, your therapist helps you identify the wrong thoughts that cause you anxiety so that you can correct them. Therapy attacks the problem from the root, not just the symptoms. In medication, your therapist prescribes drugs that can ease your symptoms. They are quick, but they can be addictive, making them the last point of call.

I have kept to the promises I made to you. I believe that reading this book has exposed you to the universal truths about anxiety disorders. You have seen that through self-care strategies, you can start to live your life to the fullest again. The best part is that these tips and strategies we've discussed are easy to practice and also very effective. Even if your symptoms are severe, I have provided you with a guide on medication and therapy. With this, you are equipped with all the knowledge you need to be free again.

My final piece of advice is that you should start seeing this as doable. You may know all the strategies that can help you, but if you don't think they will work, you will not put in the efforts that will make them work. Again, you know how effective recovery from anxiety disorders might warrant you to expose yourself to those things you fear most. Do not hesitate to do it. Find the courage to do it and reap long-term rewards.

If you can leave a favorable review, you can help me get these tips and strategies out to people who need it to be free from their fears. Thank you, and I hope you enjoyed my work.

Best wishes!

HOARDING DISORDER HELP

15 MINIMALIST STEPS TO HELP YOU DECLUTTER

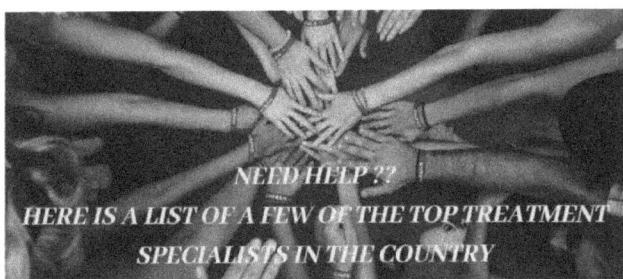

NEED HELP ??
HERE IS A LIST OF A FEW OF THE TOP TREATMENT
SPECIALISTS IN THE COUNTRY

THE LIST INCLUDES:

- *Nationally renowned treatment providers*
- *One-click linked portal access*
- *Locations and contact information*
- *Things to remember when seeking or providing help*

It's one thing to need help, and another to know where to go......

To receive your Renowned Treatment List, visit the link:

Renowned Treatment List

INTRODUCTION

"Sometimes letting things go is an act of far greater power than defending or hanging on."

— ECKHART TOLLE

If you are, or if you know, someone who has difficulty parting with literally anything and whose house is so full of clutter that it's nearly impossible to walk through, then it is quite likely the problem is a hoarding disorder. Hoarding disorder is defined as having an ongoing difficulty discarding or parting with possessions because of a perception that it is vital to save them (American Psychiatric Association, n.d.). In fact, just the thought of throwing things away can cause a hoarder significant distress. It's a real disorder that causes emotional pain and social embarrassment.

There are two things, however, to be aware of with this serious condition: First, hoarding disorder is a condition that affects millions of people. Between 2 and 5 percent of US adults suffer from this diagnosis, and up to 5 percent of the global population displays symptoms of hoarding (The Recovery Village, 2020). It's so easy for someone to think they are the only one in the world who feels this way or accumulates so much stuff, but that is far from true. Additionally, this disorder makes sufferers feel as if they are out of control of their environment. They feel helpless in the face of the clutter, and they feel ashamed, which often prevents them from seeking the help they so desperately need. But, the second thing that is important to understand about hoarding is that there is help.

To combat this serious disorder requires a solid plan for helping those affected take back control of their life. It's a process that entails manageable goals and the recognition that relief will not come all at once. It is imperative to take it one step--that is, one manageable goal--at a time. That helps better prepare them emotionally and mentally for the decluttering process. But, if you suffer from this disorder or want to help a loved one who does, where do you start? That's where my professional experience can help.

I received my doctoral degree in psychology from the University of Iowa, and I originally specialized in substance abuse. I became interested in obsessive-compulsive disorder (OCD) after my research showed an overlap between substance abuse and OCD. That led me to become a registered therapist specializing in hoarding disorder and OCD. In fact, as a clinical researcher, I have received funding from the National Institute of Mental Health to conduct research, and from that research, I have published over 150 professional, i.e., peer-reviewed, publications and book chapters on the subjects of substance abuse, OCD, and hoarding disorder. I have also worked as a consultant for hoarding task forces. Additionally, I have given lectures on the overlap between OCD and substance abuse at universities across the United States. As a result of my professional studies, I have developed a step-by-step guide to help take back control over their lives. This method is highly effective for helping any hoarder declutter their environment.

This book provides you with the tools you'll need to help yourself--or the person affected by hoarding disorder you love--to regain control and understand this challenging condition. The book describes fifteen easy-to-follow, proven steps to take to help hoarders through the declutter process. In fact, here are some of the things you'll discover in the chapters of this book:

- The #1 reason cleaning feels so difficult to do;
- How to construct a plan for decluttering success;
- How it's possible to both keep and get rid of things at the same time;
- Proven tips for managing anxiety;
- The secret to avoiding a relapse,
- How to process those feelings of shame and guilt.

And, there's more. In fact, by using the fifteen steps described in this book, it's possible to clear out as much as 80 percent of the items in the home with very little anxiety. The secrets revealed in this book provide compassionate and effective guidance to help even the most obsessive hoarder get their behaviors in check. Lastly, because everyone is their own worst critic, this book will help anyone who suffers from this condition understand the roots of hoarding and effectively declutter their environment while at the same time learning to treat themselves with compassion and patience.

You, or the loved one you watch suffer with this condition, no longer have to be ashamed of it. There is help to conquer this disorder once and for all, and you will find it in the pages of this book. The hoarding struggle is an identified disorder by professional psychologists and therapists. And, therapy does work. In fact, as much as 70 percent of patients experience positive results from therapy and are able to get their lives back on track. With the right tools, anyone can overcome this condition. It takes some time, some patience, some compassion, and a good plan. In other words, a clear strategy to take back control and rid yourself from this truly debilitating disorder. Over the course of my professional career, I have seen many success stories. I know it's possible for anyone to benefit from treatment, and I know the guidance I am providing here can help you or your loved one. I have dedicated my life to helping people with hoarding disorder reclaim their lives, and it is my sincere desire to do the same for you. There's no better time than the present to get started on your journey of healing.

I t's vital to understand the effects of hoarding disorder in order to effectively treat the condition. This overview will help explain hoarding, including the symptoms and effects, which will be helpful for identifying the disorder. The first step to successfully decluttering a home is to recognize the condition and make the decision to seek help. Here are a few of the basics to get a better understanding of hoarding disorder.

Definition of Hoarding Disorder

A hoarding disorder is identified by the acquisition of an excessive number of items which are stored chaotically in a manner that usually results in unmanageable, and often dangerous, amounts of clutter. Additionally, the items are typically of little or no monetary value.

When Does Hoarding Become a Problem?

When the clutter reaches the point where it is interfering with everyday life--for example, the person cannot get to their kitchen--or if the clutter is negatively affecting the individual's quality of life or their family's quality of life, then it has become a significant problem. An example of the latter would be if attempts to clear the clutter create significant distress and affects the familial relationships. If an individual experiences anxiety just at the thought of decluttering a space in their home, then it is interfering with their quality of life. Additionally, if family members attempt to declutter the space, the affected person may become upset, and that can cause problems with their family members. These are signals that this is more than a case of someone being a slob. If there is emotional attachment to the clutter, that indicates a hoarding disorder.

Why is Hoarding So Difficult to Treat?

One of the biggest reasons that hoarding disorder is so diffi-cult to treat is that people often don't even realize they have a problem. They frequently have very little awareness of how their behavior is affecting their life or the lives of their loved ones. Additionally, it's common for hoarders to feel shame, and that can prevent them from seeking help. Because hoarding can result in loneliness and other mental health problems, it's extremely important to encourage them to seek help, because without it, it's quite likely the problem won't resolve itself. And, it can get to the point that it poses a health and safety risk.

What Causes Hoarding Disorder?

Science has yet to fully understand the reasons why someone begins to hoard. It can be associated with other problems. For example, there is evidence that it is associated with obsessive-compulsive disorder (OCD) and obsessive-compulsive personality disorder (OCPD). It may begin with compulsive buying, the compulsive desire to get "freebies," and/or the compulsive search for perfect items. There is also evidence it is associated with severe depression, psychotic disorders such as schizophrenia, and other problems such as attention-deficit/hyperactivity disorder (ADHD). But, it could also be related to something as simple as another illness that prevents the individual from clearing out the clutter they've acquired. If, for example, someone has mobility problems and can't physically remove clutter, then it can accumulate to the point where it becomes overwhelming. Additionally, people with learning disabilities and dementia may not be able to examine the clutter, organize and categorize it, and dispose of those items they no longer need. Their condition may prevent them from being able to do those kinds of mental exercises.

Research (Tolin et al., 2018) also indicates that cognitive impairment is associated with hoarding behaviors. In one study of 83 patients diagnosed with hoarding disorder as compared to 46 healthy control participants, diagnostic interviews and measures of subjective cognitive functioning indicated that the hoarding group demonstrated more impairment than the control group. Furthermore, the degree of cognitive impairment was correlated with the severity of saving and acquiring behaviors. Cognitive impairment was further correlated with the desire to save objects in order to avoid forgetting. These results support current models that indicate decision-making deficits are at the root of hoarding behavior. Cognitive impairment disrupts decision-making skills.

Further research (Grisham & Baldwin, 2015) has sought to understand the neuropsychological underpinnings associated with hoarding disorder. Individuals who suffer from this condition are frequently reported as being easily distracted. This interferes with their ability to manage clutter through organization and by staying on task. This attention deficit was confirmed in research that examined the association of the disorder with attention deficit hyperactivity disorder (ADHD). The results of initial research were confirmed in subsequent studies, which showed more ADHD symptoms in individuals with a hoarding disorder diagnosis as compared to those participants who were healthy and those with anxiety and mood disorders. Still, other research found that those individuals with both OCD and hoarding also had symptoms of ADHD, significantly more so than those OCD patients without hoarding disorder. In those studies using neuropsychological tests to ascertain attention deficits in individuals with hoarding disorder, hoarders were found to have more difficulties than the control group with sustained and spatial attention. Though more research is necessary, there appears to be evidence for deficits in attention among hoarders.

Other research has focused on hoarders' reported desire to keep possessions in order to avoid forgetting them (Grisham & Baldwin, 2015). In fact, concern about memory was shown to be one of the strongest predictors of hoarding behavior in one study. Several studies have found that hoarders have more concern about and poorer confidence in their ability to remember the events and people in their lives. They also tend to overestimate the negative consequences of forgetting. Thus, remembering is a major concern among hoarders. But, does the research bear out their fears? In those studies of laboratory tests of memory, hoarders were, in fact, impaired in their ability to recall and copy organization on a complex figure test as compared to healthy control group participants. Hoarders also were found to have more difficulty with retaining verbal information. These results appear to offer evidence for verbal and visual memory deficits among hoarders. That strongly suggests there may be an association between memory deficits and hoarding.

Still other studies have focused on deficits in executive functioning among hoarders. Executive functioning refers to the ability of an individual to plan and make decisions. Individuals with deficits in executive functioning would have problems discarding and organizing possessions. Impairments in this regard could also be an underlying factor for poor self-regulation that is seen in those individuals with hoarding disorder. That leads to poor self-care and interpersonal deficits. As compared with OCD patients without hoarding, those with hoarding symptoms have been demonstrated to have more difficulty with initiating and completing tasks and problems associated with indecision. It's possible that task-related anxiety is interfering with these results, but hoarding patients do report difficulties in planning and executing complex, strategic motor responses and controlling interference in their efforts. That suggests problems related to self-regulation as expressed by their inability to suppress responses stimulated by a particular environment--for example, a store stimulates the need to acquire and save objects. Problems sustaining motivation for carrying out various tasks, such as discarding unused items, also reflects deficits in self-regulation. One study did find that hoarders experienced impaired decision-making abilities relative to non-hoarders, but that study was not able to be replicated. That may be due to study samples that utilize individuals with both OCD and hoarding as opposed to strictly diagnosed hoarders (Grisham & Baldwin, 2015).

Other research has examined the difficulties that hoarders have with categorization. To efficiently categorize objects, it is necessary to plan, develop grouping strategies, and make decisions related to the placement of objects in a group. Some research indicates that hoarders have a tendency to create too many, small categories, which ultimately contributes to disorganization and clutter. Hoarding participants in three studies were asked to sort personal and non-personal items into categories. The time to completion for the sorting task, the number of categories created, and the distress experienced by the participant were all measured. When compared with healthy control groups, hoarders created more piles, took longer to sort the items, and reported more distress during the process. All three investigations reported similar findings. Although there were minor discrepancies between the studies, they all support the clinical observations that hoarders have difficulty categorizing items relative to non-hoarding individuals (Grisham & Baldwin, 2015).

It's also possible that hoarding is a condition in and of itself. It is frequently associated with self-neglect. This is reflected in the fact that hoarders are more likely to live alone, be single, have experienced a neglectful or deprived childhood--i.e., they didn't have very many material things as a child or they had poor relationships with family members-- and/or have a family history of hoarding, which makes them see the clutter as normal. In the latter case, they would never have learned how to declutter; they were never taught how to prioritize and sort items in order to dispose of things they no longer need.

How Do Hoarders Perceive Their Clutter?

Many hoarders have very strong beliefs related to the need for the items they are accumulating. They might believe they will need them someday or that the item is irreplaceable for some reason. They may also associate the possession of an item with happiness or fulfillment. For that reason, any attempt to discard something can generate very strong emotions to the point where the person feels overwhelmed. That prevents them from decluttering--they simply continue to put it off or avoid actually making a decision about what can be discarded. It's also typical that the items in question are of little or no monetary value, something most people would consider rubbish. But, those afflicted with this disorder may claim these items have sentimental value or they're simply beautiful. In fact, many times they will form a strong emotional attachment to the object.

Research has shown that emotional attachments to objects is a key component of hoarding disorder. And, studies have shown that the object attachment experienced by the hoarder represents an attempt to compensate for unmet needs related to social connections. In a sample of 91 under-graduates with hoarding symptoms, object attachment was demonstrated to mediate the relationship between loneliness and hoarding behavior. And, that mediation remained consistent despite adjustments made for age and depression. That suggests that addressing issues of those unmet social connections can help lower object attachment and hoarding symptoms (Yap et al., 2020). This study highlights the importance of therapy in addressing hoarding behavior.

How Does Hoarding Differ from Collecting?

Lots of people collect things, like stamps, coins, or books, and no one thinks of them as hoarders, so what is the difference? The difference really lies in how the items are organized. Most collectors keep their collection well-organized and easily accessible. Hoarders, on the other hand, are very disorganized in their storage of the items they accumulate, and the clutter makes them largely inaccessible. For example, a collector might put newspaper clippings in a scrapbook and catalog them according to subject or time period. In contrast, a hoarder will keep large stacks of newspapers piled up throughout their entire house, which renders any specific item of interest inaccessible. The following descriptions give a better indication of the differences:

- **Collectors**: These individuals have a genuine passion for their subject of their interest. This might be stamps, antiques, model cars, and collectibles. Generally speaking, these individuals form part of a community of people with similar passions and interests. They are not isolated in their interest. They also tend to organize their collections and display them proudly for other people to see.

- **Hoarding**: In contract, because of their inability to organize their clutter, hoarders are not able to display the objects they have collected. Instead, the objects are piled up in their home in such a manner that it is difficult to find anything or even get around. Entryways are either entirely or partially blocked, and navigating from one room to another becomes difficult at best. The objects that hoarders collect also tend to have little monetary value, but despite that fact, hoarders develop an intense emotional attachment to the items they have. Because of their anxiety, depression, guilt, and shame, hoarders frequently become isolated in their homes, and are unwilling to have anyone come into their space.

What Are the Symptoms of Hoarding?

Approximately one or two people in every one hundred have serious problems with hoarding. The signs can start as early as the teen years, but they get more intense with age. While the condition can get more problematic in older age, the disorder is well-established prior to that time. The symptoms typically include any or all of the following:

- An inability to discard possessions, often accompanied by an intense emotional attachment to the items in the home;
- Keeping or collecting large amounts of objects with little or no monetary value--for example, junk mail, newspapers, magazines, or items that the person intends to repair or reuse;
- Anxiety when attempting to clean or clear things out;
- Difficulty organizing or categorizing possessions;

- Indecisiveness regarding how to store things;
- Difficulty managing daily tasks like cooking, cleaning, or paying bills;
- General distress;
- Suspicion of anyone who touches your possessions;
- Poor or deteriorating relationships with family or friends;
- Obsessive thoughts and actions;
- Functional impairments;
- Clutter blindness.

Additionally, psychologists have identified some typical patterns seen with hoarding. Specifically, there are three identified patterns, referred to as hoarding life cycle patterns.

Hoarding Life Cycle Pattern #1

This pattern is identified by a person who can, in fact, regularly decide about discarding items, but develops a problem through the extreme acquisition of objects. In this case, the clutter can be brought under temporary control, but it will recur with the arrival of newly acquired items. In this pattern, there is an ebb and flow to the clutter that is dependent upon the number of items arriving versus those that are being discarded at any given point. The individual is able to give items away to people they know will appreciate the object, use it, and take good care of it. If this individual experiences some kind of destabilizing setback that upsets the checks and balances created by regularly discarding items, the clutter can significantly increase to levels where the individual feels overwhelmed. Such setbacks are ultimately inevitable.

Hoarding Life Cycle Pattern #2

This pattern is one where discarding items occurs infrequently, but so do acquisitions. Both occur at lower rates, and thus, the hoarding pattern takes longer to develop into a serious clutter problem. Still, the potential is there, and the situation will ultimately result in extreme clutter. This pattern is associated with object acquisition, rigid saving, and a focus on the possibility of using the item. These kinds of hoarders want to get the most value from the items they collect. They compare the price of the item with the use they get out of it. If they don't believe they have gotten their money's worth out of the item, they are unwilling to let it go. They equate keeping the item with somehow retaining the money they spent on it. Even if the item proves not to be as useful as they had anticipated, they still compare the money spent on the item's ideal value. Thus, keeping the item makes them feel as if they are getting their money out of it, even if it is only rarely used.

With this pattern, discarding items also happens differently. These hoarders will tell themselves that they are too busy to take the time to discard the item. They may, in fact, have genuinely busy lives, but though they tell themselves they will do it later, they never seem to find the time. They over-commit their time and energy in a way that they are over-scheduled, which is but another symptom of compulsive behavior. Why are they keeping themselves so busy? This is an attempt to provide a justification for failing to face the problems their behavior is generating. They too are vulnerable to setbacks that can significantly and rapidly increase the clutter build up in their homes.

Hoarding Life Cycle Pattern #3

This pattern involves individuals who don't accumulate much more than the average person, but they never discard anything. Nothing that enters their home will ever leave it. They might have a recycling system, but somehow the items they collect never make into the recycle bin. They may also claim to be storing and saving items for others--a younger sibling's children, for example--but they never actually donate those items to the intended recipient. This offers the individual a noble cause as justification for their hoarding. It might take a while, but this will ultimately result in an extreme clutter situation. It's a particularly intractable pattern since the individual claims to be doing it for other people.

What Kinds of Things Do People Typically Hoard?

People can hoard many different types of things, but there are some common patterns with regard to what people most frequently tend to hoard. The following is a list of some of the more common items that people hoard:

- Newspapers and magazines;
- Books;
- Bills and receipts:
- Containers like plastic bags and cardboard boxes;
- Household supplies;
- Clothes;
- Leaflets and letters, including junk mail.

While these are the more common items that people hoard, there are other things as well. For example, hoarders might collect animals, which they frequently don't care for properly. Recent data also shows that some people hoard huge amounts of electronic data and emails that they don't want to delete.

Why is Hoarding Disorder a Problem?

There are several reasons hoarding is a problem. First, it can completely take over a person's life. Their excessive clutter can become so overwhelming that they can have trouble even getting around their house. It can affect their work performance, personal hygiene, and their relationships. Hoarders often feel shame because of their disorder, and that frequently makes them reluctant or unable to have visitors. They don't even want to allow a repairman into their house for essential repairs. And, all of this can cause isolation and profound loneliness. Furthermore, the excessive clutter can pose a health risk to anyone living in or visiting the house. The clutter can make cleaning difficult, which in turn leads to unhygienic conditions that can result in rat or insect infestations. Moreover, the chaotic storage poses a fire risk and can block the exits. The clutter also makes it easy to trip and fall, and if the stacks of items are high enough, the clutter can even fall on anyone in the house, causing serious injuries. All of this adds up to a very serious problem.

What to Do If You Suspect Someone is Hoarding

It can be very distressing to watch someone you love succumb to this disorder. And, if they don't realize they have a problem, it can be very difficult to convince them to seek help. But, that's exactly what you should do. Be sensitive about the issue as you explain your concerns for their well-being. It's also important to reassure them that no one will be going into their homes and throwing anything away. Explain that therapy involves empowering them to conquer their disorder and a doctor can help explain the options for how to accomplish that. It's best to seek a referral to someone who is familiar with hoarding disorder and any associated conditions like OCD. Whatever you do, you don't want to call someone in to clean the clutter. That can cause more problems than it solves.

How are Hoarding Disorders Treated?

Treating a hoarding disorder is difficult even when the patient realizes they have a problem and wants to solve it. One of the main treatments is called cognitive-behavioral therapy or CBT. With this type of therapy, the therapist helps the person get at the root of their disorder. To truly conquer the problem, people affected with this condition have to understand the underlying psychological reasons for the behavior. It works by changing how the person thinks (cognitive) and acts (behavior). To do that, the therapist will explore how the patient thinks about themselves, the world, and other people. Moreover, the therapy helps the patient understand how they think about these things affects their thoughts and feelings.

While CBT therapy sessions occur over a long period of time, they are often also accompanied by "homework." They also frequently include sessions in the patient's home where the therapist will help them work on the clutter. It's important to be patient since the therapy typically lasts for months before the ultimate goal is achieved. And, the goal is not simply to declutter the home; the goal is to help the person overcome the psychological reasons behind the hoarding behavior and help them improve their decision-making and organizational skills.

It's also important to reassure the patient that a therapist won't throw anything away; rather, their goal is to help the person regain control over their own life, to identify and challenge any underlying beliefs that are behind the problem. As the patient is able to start discarding items in their home, they understand that nothing bad has happened and that they are becoming better at organizing the items in their home. With that for encouragement, they will have more motivation to continue working on the problem. By the time the patient has finished the treatment, they will have a much better understanding of their own behavior, and they will have a plan to avoid relapsing into more hoarding in the future. It is also possible that the therapist may elect to administer antidepressant medications. These include medicines called selective serotonin reuptake inhibitors (SSRIs). These medications prevent a buildup of serotonin on nerve receptor cells in the brain. A buildup of serotonin is associated with depression.

In sum, it's evident that this condition is far more complex than simply shoddy housekeeping. The effects of the disorder are serious and sometimes dangerous. If you're reading this book, you likely understand that either you're a hoarder or someone you love is. If, as a hoarder, you're not seeking treatment, the first step is to find a therapist with experience in treating hoarding disorder and seek help. It's an important part of getting to the root of the disorder. If you're already receiving treatment, then this book is a useful tool with decluttering tips you can use to support your treatment.

For anyone serious about changing their life, they have to treat this disorder like they would any other illness. They must seek professional help, and use other sources, such as this book, to help overcome the challenges that they encounter on the path to healthy living.

Chapter Summary

In this chapter, hoarding disorder has been defined and described. Specifically, the following topics have been covered:

- The definition of hoarding disorder;
- The signs of hoarding disorder--compulsive collection of items and chaotic organization;
- Associated conditions with hoarding disorder;

- How the individual views their clutter;
- The typical treatment for hoarding disorder;
- What to do if you suspect someone you know is a hoarder.

The next chapter will focus on recognizing how important ongoing support and therapy is for the treatment of hoarding disorder.

H oarding disorder can be a difficult condition to treat, because often, people don't really understand the negative impact of this problem on their health and their lives. For that reason, they frequently don't believe they need any kind of treatment. This is particularly true if the items or animals that the person hoards offer them psychological comfort. That makes it difficult for them to think about losing those items or animals, and if someone suggests they should get rid of them, they will often react emotionally, becoming very angry or expressing frustration.

Insight Problems

Many researchers believe part of the problem in recognizing the need for help is a lack of insight into the severity of their symptoms and the need for change. In fact, studies have shown that people with obsessive-compulsive disorder who hoard have worse insight into their own symptoms of hoarding than people with OCD who do not hoard (Owen, 2020). And, that lack of insight causes significant problems that include avoiding seeking help, withdrawing early from treatment, and/or failing to comply with the homework assignments given by the therapist. Moreover, it is this lack of insight that frustrates family members and friends, and can eventually drive them away. Frequently, the only way that people finally agree to seek treatment is after they have been threatened with some negative consequence like eviction or divorce. They may enter therapy to prevent the negative consequence rather than because they believe they need help. That is precisely why treatment is often ineffective.

Once they do accept that they need some kind of help, it is important for them and their family to realize that recovery from a condition as complicated as hoarding disorder doesn't occur overnight, and it is an ongoing process. It is something you deal with on a daily basis. For that reason, asking for help is imperative as part of the process of treating this condition. There are a number of therapeutic options, but the most common psychological therapeutic choice is cognitive-behavioral therapy (CBT).

Cognitive Behavioral Therapy

Cognitive-behavioral therapy has shown great promise for treating hoarding disorder. Research (International OCD Foundation, 2020) indicates that some 70 to 80 percent of individuals with hoarding disorder show significant improvement after nine to twelve months of treatment with CBT.

This type of therapy helps people affected with this disorder get at the root of their condition; in other words, it helps them get at the psychological reasons behind their compulsion. But, that's not all CBT does. It will also help teach a patient strategies for preventing further hoarding behavior and decluttering their home. Furthermore, it helps to reduce their anxiety as they declutter their home, and it helps with organization and decision-making. Additionally, it helps hoarders to identify and challenge those persistent thoughts and beliefs that they have regarding acquiring and saving various items. It also teaches them how to resist the urge to acquire more items. More specifically, the following topics are what patients undergoing CBT will learn about and experience:

- **How to process information:** Part of the problem is that they have difficulty making decisions regarding what kinds of possessions they need, what to keep, and how to organize what they do have. Thus, treatment focuses on generating and enhancing skills associated with sorting, organizing, and decision-making.

- **Emotional attachment to possessions:** Many hoarders have intense sentimental attachments to the items they hoard. They are very reluctant to even consider discarding them. For that reason, CBT therapists will use techniques such as cognitive restructuring and exposure therapy to help challenge those beliefs. This will help the patient to explore the truth about the objects and their value as well as the consequences associated with keeping or discarding them.

Cognitive restructuring involves learning to identify and dispute irrational thoughts as well as negative automatic thoughts through the use of techniques like guided questioning, recording, and disputation. Basically, hoarders learn to test their ideas for accuracy before simply accepting them as true. The idea is to replace those thoughts that generate anxiety with more rational, positive thoughts that help reduce anxiety.

- **Beliefs about possessions**: Hoarders have intense beliefs about their possessions that they must maintain control over them. They feel that they have a responsibility to see that the item doesn't go to waste. For that reason, CBT focuses on restructuring those beliefs by critically examining their validity.

- **Behavioral Avoidance**: One of the problems that hoarders have is in coping with situations that generate anxiety. That anxiety is what causes them to avoid having to deal with the situation, something they have been doing as the items have been piling up in their home. CBT teaches them how to not only face what feels initially like an overwhelming situation in a systematic manner, but also to develop different strategies for anxiety-producing situations. A CBT therapist will help the patient replace their avoidance with adaptive coping strategies that they can use throughout their life as difficult situations arise.

The therapy ideally involves regular home visits as well as visits to settings where clients are triggered in their hoarding behavior, for example, flea markets, yard sales, and shopping centers. Additionally, the therapy rotates its focus among the behaviors of acquiring items, sorting and organizing materials, and discarding unnecessary, redundant, or useless items. The progression of the therapy depends on individual circumstances--some find decluttering is the best first goal and tolerate the stress that brings while others find it easier to first get control over acquiring behaviors.

The progress made by patients being treated for hoarding disorder depends in part on the ability of the individual to change their thinking. The goal is to reduce the emotional distress associated with losing possessions. To help an individual change their thinking, clinicians may employ discussion and CBT methods. CBT therapy typically progresses in the following stages:

Assessment: This is the stage where the clinician will assess the specific symptoms including how they interfere with everyday life, the safety problems they might cause, and any physical or other mental health issues that might affect treatment.

Formulation of a Personal Model of Hoarding Behavior: At this point, a therapist will work with the patient to ensure they understand the causes of hoarding disorder and how their own symptoms have developed into a serious problem. They will explain the causal factors, such as psychological vulnerabilities, problems processing infor-

mation, and the beliefs and emotions associated with the importance of objects. From there, the therapist and patient can begin the process of gaining insight into how these factors have contributed to excessive acquisition and saving that has resulted in the significant build-up of clutter.

Motivational Interviewing: These are techniques that help patients to consider how their hoarding behaviors fit within their own value system and the goals they have for their life. These will help to sustain a patient's motivation for change.

Excessive Acquisition Reduction: While patients may be initially directed to avoid situations where acquisition behaviors are triggered, the focus of this part of CBT is to gradually expose the individual to those situations that act as triggers for their hoarding behaviors. Examples include driving to a store, but not going in, then going in, but not touching anything, and then picking up items, but not buying them. This kind of practice can help the patient develop strategies to resist the urge to acquire more objects and then they can progress to more challenging situations.

Skills Training: Hoarders typically have difficulty processing information, and that leads to significant skill deficits. They might, for example, have difficulty staying focused on tasks, have problems organizing items into logical categories, or have little ability to plan ahead to achieve their goals or solve basic problems. This kind of training will help them to develop those important skills, which will give them a healthy foundation for resisting hoarding urges.

Practicing Letting Go: This gives the individual the skills they need to part with their possessions. Typically, they will be encouraged to work from easier to harder items and make decisions about which to keep and which to let go. This is part of exposure therapy and it provides them with an opportunity to learn tolerance for the negative emotions that arise and to challenge those negative feelings to better understand and deal with them.

Therapy for Hoarding Beliefs: Throughout the treatment process, patients are encouraged to be mindful of their thoughts and feelings about acquiring and discarding possessions. This part of the therapy will help them explore those dysfunctional beliefs regarding the future usefulness of objects, concerns they have about waste, sentimental attachments, and the need to keep their memories alive. Therapists work with their patients to help them develop questions regarding the possessions in order to better evaluate the accuracy of their thinking. There are a number of methods that therapists use to help patients challenge their beliefs and consider alternative behaviors as they come to understand those beliefs are not realistic.

Relapse Prevention: As patients make progress with their hoarding behaviors, it is important that they develop good habits to replace the hoarding habits. Clinicians work with their patients in this regard. The good habits include things like putting things away immediately after they are brought into the home, cleaning up immediately after a meal or other activity, removing trash and recycling on a regular basis, and addressing those particularly difficult situations that vary between individuals. Therapists work with their patients to ensure they have developed good habits to meet the challenges that will surely arise in the months after treatment comes to an end.

In cases where anxiety is undermining progress, it is also possible that a therapist might prescribe medication. The medications frequently used for hoarding disorder include antidepressants like venlafaxine and paroxetine, but it is imperative that medication be given in conjunction with CBT. These types of medications are known as selective serotonin reuptake inhibitors (SSRIs). Serotonin is a neuro-chemical that is known to be associated with depression. As neurons--nerve cells in the brain--communicate with one another, neurochemicals like serotonin facilitate that process by bridging the gap between the nerve cells. The gap is called a synapse and serotonin crosses the gap and lands on a receptor cell on the other side of the synapse. There it accumulates until it is recycled. Normally, the brain takes care of this without help, but if there is any problem with that process, it can result in too much serotonin accumulation or too little. And, that can cause problems like depression or anxiety. Thus, if they're suffering from depression or anxiety, a CBT therapist might decide to prescribe one of these medications.

Supportive Relationships

As part of the healing process, it is vital to include family and friends, and CBT can sometimes involve family/relationship therapy. The support of family is critical to helping a hoarder as they confront difficult emotions and thoughts and learn how to change those negative patterns into productive, positive behaviors. The family's support can help inspire the afflicted person to continue making progress in their treatment and to persevere on the journey to healthy behaviors. For children with hoarding disorder, the parents are an important element in their treatment. In fact, parents often have to learn how to change their behaviors since they likely contributed to the problem in a process often called, "family accommodation." It's easy for them to think they are helping to alleviate their child's anxiety by allowing them to acquire and save the items they hoard. In fact, the opposite is true as the hoarding serves to increase anxiety. That's why it's important for the entire family to be engaged in the treatment process.

Ongoing Treatment

It is important to recognize that hoarding disorder is a very challenging issue. It is difficult to treat and recovery can take a long time. The ongoing support and therapy a hoarder receives from a professional cognitive behavioral therapy counselor as well as the support of family and friends are crucial for helping them persevere in the decluttering process. It's important to recognize when you make progress in this fight. Even small steps should be applauded, but it's also important to recognize that the treatment for hoarding disorder is an ongoing process that requires continued support to work through the significant problems associated with this disorder.

Chapter Summary

This chapter has covered the importance of seeking help and continuing supportive therapy throughout the decluttering process and beyond. Specifically, the following topics were covered:

- The difficulty with treating hoarding disorder;
- The insight problems most hoarders experience;

- Cognitive Behavioral Therapy (CBT) and how it can help;
- The adaptive coping strategies hoarders learn with CBT;
- The importance of supportive relationships.

The next chapter will discuss how to take control by setting goals and planning.

I t's important at this stage to discuss a little about goal setting and planning in general. There are a few simple things to remember no matter what the ultimate goal is, but this is also particularly relevant for decluttering in response to a hoarding disorder. It's important to be systematic when approaching the problem. Take it one step at a time and it will be far easier to achieve the desired goals.

Tip #1: Identify the Problem

It is important to understand the nature of the problem. It's a good start to answer the following questions:

- How is the clutter affecting their life?
- How will their life change when the home is decluttered?

- How do they feel about the clutter?
- How will they feel with the clutter gone?
- Do they avoid having people over because of the clutter?
- Will they have more of a social life when the clutter is gone?
- Is the clutter affecting their relationships?
- Will their relationships improve when the clutter is gone?

By answering these questions, the individual can identify the specific problem and the positive benefits that will result once the problem is resolved. It's good to have a clear understanding of the problem and write that down in order to see it in black and white. That will also help for tracking progress.

Tip #2: Define the Ultimate Goal

Ideally, this will involve more than simply cleaning or decluttering the home. It should also involve goals in other areas of life, like improvements in relationships or the ability to be more social. In a sense, this involves describing in detail what success looks like. For example, this might sound like, "When I have decluttered my home, I will happily invite people over for social events, I will feel like I live in a clean and safe environment, and I will have a beautifully organized home." It's important to be as specific as possible so that when the goal has been achieved, it will look as envisioned. Also, by stating specific goals, it's helpful for staying motivated and on course.

Tip #3: Create a Vision Board

The next important thing to do before actually starting with the decluttering process is to create a vision board that visually displays the reasons for decluttering. These are taken from the ultimate goals described in Tip #2. It's helpful to visually represent those goals, and that includes more than simply a clean, well-organized home. That should be on the board too, but so should how it will *feel* to have a decluttered home. For example, a vision board for this process could contain happy pictures of oneself as well as family and friends. It's also a good idea to include pictures of tidy shelves and cupboards as well as pictures that represent being able to easily find things. Posting inspirational quotes on the vision board is also helpful for motivation. And, when there are moments of doubt or when the anxiety levels rise too high, examining the vision board can help to calm an individual and get them back on track.

To create a vision board, the following items are required:

- Some kind of board--it could be a cork board or poster board, although it might be more helpful to have a board where it's possible to pin items to and move them around.

- Scissors, tape, pins, or glue to affix pictures to the board.

- Magazines from which images and quotes can be cut.

- Photographs of happy family and friends.

- Time--most people need about an hour or two to put together a vision board. It should be a stress-free activity since this will be a source of inspiration and motivation. Therefore, it's important to make sure to allow for enough time to get it just right.

The vision board is something that they will look to regularly for inspiration, so it should be placed in a prominent location in the home where it can be seen easily.

Tip #4: Make a Map of the Home

Now that the long-term, general goals have been identified, it's time to examine the home and break down the declutter process into a series of short-term, specific goals. This begins by making a map of the home. Each space in the home should be examined, and areas within each space should be identified for processing. This will be important for prioritizing areas for clearing the clutter.

Tip #5: Grade the Clutter

Once the map of the home has been made and the areas of focus identified, it is now time to grade the clutter. Use a scale of 1 - 3, with 1 being the least cluttered and 3 being the most cluttered. This will make it possible to identify the areas that will take the most work to clear, and that will help with prioritization when planning the work.

Tip #6: Plan the Work

It's critical that when planning the work, it be broken down into manageable goals. If not, the task will simply seem overwhelming and there will be an urge to abandon the plan and relapse into hoarding. Remember the adage, "How do you eat an elephant? One bite at a time." By breaking the decluttering process down into a series of small, easily achievable goals, it will help to not only achieve those goals, but to stay inspired and motivated. Additionally, those small goals can be celebrated when they've been achieved.

As part of the planning process, the grades assigned to each space should be used to prioritize areas for addressing. It's also a good idea to identify spaces within each room for priority work. Start by identifying those short-term goals--areas for decluttering--that can be achieved within a short period of time. For example, perhaps you have identified a closet within the most cluttered room to clean first. That's something that may take a week to break down the clutter, but at the end of that week, that clean closet is something to celebrate. And, that builds much-needed motivation.

By identifying a series of small areas that represent short term goals, it's possible to build a plan for the work. Mark each area on the map of the home in order of priority. It's also a good idea as part of the plan to state how the goals will be accomplished. That will be discussed in more detail in a later chapter, but suffice it to say here that it's important to have a system in place that you can follow with the least amount of uncertainty regarding how to accomplish the goals. That's particularly important for a hoarder since the urge to give up is a frequent problem.

It's also a good idea to make note on the plan of longer-term goals. These can include things like decluttering an entire room, then an entire section of the home (for example, the upstairs), and finally, the decluttering of the entire house itself.

Tip #7: Write Everything Down

Writing everything down is a good way to ensure that you follow the plan. It's easy to get off-track if nothing is written down in black and white. In fact, there are a number of psychological benefits to writing everything down. They include the following:

- **Positive emotions:** Whether writing about stressors or goals, writing things down can create a happier, more positive attitude. For the person affected by this disorder, writing things down helps develop self-discipline for following the plan and decluttering each space, it helps with problem-solving when deciding what to do with the hoarded items, and it helps to alleviate anxiety. All of these benefits lead to more positive emotions.

- **Clarity**: When you have a written plan, it alleviates the stress of having to make decisions. The decision is made, and it's in the plan. The goals, priorities, and intentions behind the decluttering process are clear and easily accessible. That makes it easier to actually tackle the work.

- **Documentation**: Writing everything down helps document the process, the intent behind the work, and it helps keep track of the progress.

- **Sense of accomplishment**: By writing out the plan, it will be easier to document accomplishments. And, there will be something to mark off the list, which helps create a sense of satisfaction with a job well done.

- **Boosts efficiency**: Having a written plan eliminates the need to decide what to do on any given day. The plan has it all laid out. That helps to get going on the work quickly, and in that way, it boosts efficiency.

Tip #8: Set a Start Date

With a written plan and work priorities identified, it is important to set a start date. A plan is great, but if it never gets initiated, it doesn't do much good. By setting a date to start the work, it will create motivation even as it allows for necessary preparation. Subsequent chapters will discuss allotting a specific time frame for each task in your plan as well as the general start and end date for the work. This will help eliminate any procrastination as well.

With these 8 basic tips, it's possible to create a plan for action. It's important to remember a few things. First, be realistic about the difficulty in achieving each goal and the time it will take to do so. It's also important to involve other people in the process. They will help establish a sense of accountability as well as support and encouragement. They are, in effect, a source of motivation. And, they can help to alleviate the anxiety that may arise during the decluttering process.

Another important concept to include in any decluttering plan is a way and time to evaluate progress. Perhaps, it is done on a weekly basis whereby they would consult the map and see how many of the identified goals for the week were actually achieved. If all of them were achieved, that's something to celebrate, and it should be celebrated. For that, it's important to establish a system of rewards. Rewards might include going to dinner at a nice restaurant or a favorite activity. It's probably a good idea to avoid rewards that would require accumulating more objects. Instead, go someplace fun or do something fun, but in any case, be sure to reward those goals that have been successfully achieved. If some of the goals were not achieved, celebrate the ones that were and tweak the plan. Don't get discouraged and give up just because some goals were not met. Keep going and pretty soon, all of the goals will be achieved. By celebrating the accomplishments achieved, that will provide more motivation to keep going.

Chapter Summary

This chapter discussed how to take control of the declutter process through setting goals and planning. Specifically, the following topics were discussed:

- Being systematic in the approach to setting goals and planning the work;
- Identifying the problem and describing success;
- Creating a vision board for inspiration;
- Making a map of the home and prioritizing the work;

- Planning the work, writing everything down, and setting a start date;
- Tracking progress and rewarding achievements.

The next chapter will present information on designing a schedule and managing time.

A t this stage, they have created a plan for decluttering their home and identified a start date. The next step in the decluttering process is to create a schedule for the time frame for achieving each decluttering goal. This time frame should ideally include plenty of time for each task, and allow for taking it one small space at a time. It's also important to remember that sometimes a task will take longer than anticipated, so build a little cushion into the schedule. If a particular task takes even longer than the allotted time with the cushion, it's critical not to use that as a punishment or to think of it as failure. As long as they don't give up, they won't fail.

Begin with the Map

The map of the house with the identified prioritized areas will help to design a schedule for the decluttering process. Begin by choosing between one and three prioritized areas. Assign dates to each area for decluttering. Be sure to be reasonable about the time frame needed to declutter each room. Not doing so will set them up for failure and can be discouraging. It's also important to understand that it's unlikely that an entire room will be decluttered within one span of time. It's much better to break the room down into smaller spaces. For example, if the first space is a bedroom, that can be broken down into the following areas: closet, dresser drawers, bedside tables, and any other storage areas like a trunk at the end of the bed, or a storage container under the bed. Also, if things are piled on the floor, then be sure to include floor space, which can also be broken down into separate spaces, e.g., floor space to the right of the bed, floor space to the left of the bed, and floor space in front of the bed.

How much time is needed to declutter an entire space depends on several factors. These include whether you have the entire day to devote to the project, only a few hours in the evening after work, how much clutter is present, how large the space is, and whether or not difficult emotions arise that slow the progress. It's a good idea to allot more time than might be necessary for a space so as to avoid feelings of failure or discouragement. If there's a lot of clutter and only a few hours a day that can be devoted to the decluttering process, then a small space could take anywhere from one to three weeks. The amount of time it takes to fully declutter a space is not as important as consistent progress. For planning purposes, set a time frame that is much more than you think you'll need.

The Pomodoro Technique

More important than the overall time frame is the work time devoted to decluttering a single space. The Pomodoro Technique is a popular time management technique invented in the 1990s by Francesco Cirillo. The technique is named for the tomato-shaped timer Cirillo used to track his work as a student. It's a helpful technique for breaking down any large task or series of tasks into short, timed intervals that will help to boost efficiency. It also trains the brain to stay focused during those short intervals and it improves attention span and concentration skills. The technique is cyclical in that work is accomplished in short sprints followed by regular breaks. That helps ensure consistent productivity, and the breaks bolster motivation and creativity.

To demonstrate how the technique works, imagine the task is decluttering a table. To start, set a timer for 25 minutes and work on the decluttering until the timer rings. When the timer rings, take a 5 minute break before beginning a second 25-minute interval. This results in enhanced concentration during the work period, which in turn, reduces the overall time needed for the task. In that way, it helps dramatically improve efficiency. This technique can be applied to decluttering each space within each area of the house, and it will help to reduce the time it takes to entirely declutter the home.

The Two Minute Rule

This is another method for increasing productivity that was designed by consultant David Allen. It helps form new habits and complete tasks by breaking them down into small steps. Again, imagine the table to be decluttered--begin with some action that takes no more than two minutes. Perhaps, start by collecting papers into a pile or clearing away coffee mugs--either of those is something that can be completed within two minutes. Keep track of the time to ensure you're accomplishing these micro-goals within the two minute time period. This technique produces an enhanced sense of accomplishment because it's possible to achieve a goal within a very short period of time. That motivates them to keep going and it generates a long list of accomplishments in a very short period of time. That makes the overall goal of decluttering the entire home seem much more achievable. This rule will also help to prevent procrastination, because after all, the job only requires two minutes. And then, it seems much easier to take on another two minute job, and then another. Once one job is started, it's easier to keep going. That's how this method increases productivity.

Set Schedules for Each Task in Each Space

It's important not to try to do too much at once. By approaching the entire decluttering process one task at a time rather than thinking about the whole thing, it will help keep you focused on goal-oriented tasks. While it's important to set a schedule for each task, it's also important to be flexible. There are a number of things that can delay the process, which makes it difficult to judge the time required for each area or even each space within the areas. Some tasks will take longer than expected, and sometimes, challenging emotions and thoughts will arise during the process. It's important to address those as they arise since that is an important part of the healing process. Self-compassion is a crucial part of confronting those difficult emotions, and it's also acceptable to adjust the schedule as the need arises. The most important part of the decluttering process is to keep going, to make constant progress. The overall time frame is not something that is set in stone, but continuous progress is critical.

Chapter Summary

This chapter discussed the importance of setting a time frame for the decluttering process. Specifically, the following topics were covered:

- Using the map to assign time frames to each area of the house;
- The Pomodoro Technique for increasing efficiency by breaking down large tasks into smaller ones;
- The two minute rule to increase productivity by taking on tasks that take less than two minutes;
- Setting schedules for each task, but remaining flexible and practicing self-compassion.

The next chapter presents information on creating a system for decluttering.

STEP 5: CREATE A SORTING SYSTEM AND PREPARE YOUR RESOURCES

B eing fully prepared is an important part of the decluttering process. It will help them feel organized and give them a system to follow so that when they begin, they won't be distracted by constant delays created by the need for more supplies.

Create an Organization System

Before it is possible to effectively declutter your home, it's important to devise an organization system. Decluttering will be difficult since there is likely a long history of finding it impossible to throw things away. By devising a plan, it will help to know what to do when faced with the clutter. A useful organization system is what's called the "Four Box Method." This method involves preparing four containers to use during the declutter process for each area of the house. They should be clearly labeled with "throw away," "donate/sell," "storage," and "put away." The creation of these boxes alone can generate anxious feelings, but they must remember that they are the one who is in control. If they struggle with the idea of throwing things away or donating or selling them, return to the vision board and remind them of exactly why they're doing this.

The Four Box Method

The four box method helps to keep the decluttering process moving along. It prevents the need to figure out what to do with the items that you're not keeping. As mentioned, the idea is to create four boxes for each area of the house to be decluttered:

- **Throw Away:** This box is for any item identified as unnecessary and not worth selling or donating. Donation centers often require that items be in good condition, and if an item's not in good enough condition to donate, it is probably also not in good enough condition to sell. That only leaves discarding it if it is not an item that you're keeping.
- **Donate/Sell:** This presents an opportunity to be generous and think about the uses someone else

might have use for the item. If it is something that isn't really being used, then it's preferable to make it available to others who might find more uses for it. Additionally, it could provide them with a financial benefit if they're able to sell it.

- **Storage:** This box is for things that they can't part with but also don't need regularly. Because you'll be keeping these items, it's important to organize them well. That means making an inventory of the items in the box, and storing that inventory with the box or writing it on the outside. That way, should the need for an item in this box arise, it will be easy to find. It's also a good idea to group similar items together. For example, any items associated with the kitchen can be grouped in the kitchen storage box or out of season clothing can be put in one box.

- **Put Away:** This should be the smallest category, and it should contain only those items that will be out on a regular basis. A good way to check for that is to first determine a place where each item will go. If there is something that doesn't have a place, that might indicate it belongs in another box. If they end up with too many of these items, to avoid cluttering your home again, then it will be

necessary to reassess their importance. Revisit the
vision board to remember all of the goals for the
project and the reasons behind those goals.

Once the four box system is in place, it is then possible to
declutter according to category. Begin with items that have
little sentimental value and that are clearly trash. From
there, it is possible to move on to the category of items that
are identified as no longer useful, but that aren't rubbish.
These are for donations or to sell. Then, move on to the
materials to store and those that you will keep. Just because
they've moved on to a different category doesn't mean there
won't be more items for that box. But, by decluttering the
area by category, it is possible to eliminate the majority of
items in the space that belong in that box. And, it will be
possible to organize the materials in a space at a higher level.
For example, begin with trash versus not trash, then
donate/sell versus keep, and finally, store versus use regularly. In this way, the process of decluttering will be much
more efficient. Finally, be sure to make an inventory of the
contents of each box. It might be a wise idea to buy labels for
this purpose.

Gather Supplies

Once the organizational system is ready, it's time to get resources in the form of cleaning supplies. Here's a list of some of the supplies necessary for cleaning and decluttering:

- Heavy-duty trash bags;
- Empty boxes;
- A mop;
- A bucket;
- Disinfectant spray;
- Cleaning cloths;
- A dustpan;
- A broom;
- A vacuum cleaner;
- A step ladder;
- A shovel, particularly if the home is extremely cluttered.

It's important to be aware that simply gathering supplies might trigger hoarding behavior, and that can result in an excess of materials. That will just add to the problem, so it might be a good idea to enlist the help of family and friends to get these supplies. Provide them with a list of supplies, and they can make sure to get just what is needed and no more. That will prevent triggering hoarding behavior while buying supplies.

It's also likely that the decluttering process will result in an enormous amount of rubbish to be discarded. It might be a good idea to arrange for a skip/dumpster bin to be delivered to the front of the house. That will help ensure that once rubbish is identified, it can be discarded immediately before there is time to rethink the decision. It will also prevent simply moving the items to a different part of the house where they become part of a separate clutter pile.

By creating an organizational system, such as the four box method, it will be much easier to declutter any space. It will also reduce the amount of thought process involved in deciding what to do with an item. Gathering supplies will help in the preparation so that there will be no reason to delay decluttering any more. At this point, they have a plan, a time frame, and an organizational system for decluttering their home. It's time to get to work!

Chapter Summary

This chapter presented information about a good organizational system, the four box method, as well as the materials needed for decluttering any space. Specifically, the following topics were covered:

- The four box method;
- What goes in each of the four boxes--trash, donate/sell, storage, and put away;

- The supplies needed for decluttering;
- What to do to avoid hoarding behavior while gathering supplies;
- Disposing of rubbish immediately by using a skip/dumpster bin.

The next chapter will present information on decluttering one small area at a time.

STEP 6: TACKLE ONE SMALL AREA AT A TIME

O nce a plan is in place and the supplies have been gathered, it's time to begin the decluttering work. If the job is big and help is required, be sure to have a family member or friend on hand for help and support, or hire an assistant for the day. It might also be a good idea to make lunch before beginning so that taking a break is easier to do. When it's time to get to work, here is how to proceed:

Start with the Map

Begin with a small area on the map. It should be a high priority area, but it's best to begin in an area with minimal items that have sentimental value. The bathroom is a good choice to tackle first. It's less likely to have items of sentimental value and it's an area that's regularly used, so when it's clean, it will engender a sense of achievement every time it's used. Beginning with areas of low sentimental value is helpful until the person has acclimated to the process. Once the process is well-established, it will be easier to tackle those areas that will cause more challenging emotions to arise. When the area on the map is identified, choose a small space within the area to begin. Remember to use the two-minute rule and the Pomodoro Technique as you proceed.

Select a Space within the Map Area

Once the area is selected, choose a space within the area to begin the actual decluttering process. For example, if they select the bathroom to begin, start with the cabinets under the sink. Another small space in the bathroom would be the medicine cabinet. These small areas will be easier to declutter, thereby providing a sense of accomplishment as that small goal is successfully achieved.

Stage the Belongings

Before they begin the actual work of staging, set a timer to work for 25 minutes of uninterrupted work--the Pomodoro Technique. Within that 25 minute time period, divide the tasks into two-minute jobs. For example, one two-minute job in the medicine cabinet might be removing and dividing the expired medication from the current medication.

Once the timer is set and the two-minute jobs identified, begin working by staging the belongings. That means remove them from where they are stored or piled to an area where it's possible to see them clearly. This can add a shock value to the process. Hoarders are often not aware of just how much stuff they've accumulated. This technique is also useful for revealing duplicates of items. Once the items are staged, it's easier to identify what is trash, what can be donated or sold, and what needs to be put away or stored.

When staging the belongings, they can be divided into categories if there are different types of items. For example, if the space is that medicine cabinet in the bathroom, perhaps there are current medications, expired medications, makeup materials, dental floss, and band-aids in the cabinet. Separate the items by type to better identify what and how many of each are present. As already mentioned for this example, one way to divide medications is by expiration date--those which are expired versus those which are current.

Declutter by Category

Now that everything is staged, it will be easier to see what and how many items are present. This will make it easier to further divide the items into the four box categories of trash, donate/sell, store, or put away. Begin by removing the items in the trash category. Once the trash box is full, take it out to the skip/dumpster bin and empty it immediately. If this presents a problem for the individual, have the family or friend assisting them do this or accompany them to the dumpster. Then, move on to the donate/sell category and put those items in their box. Place the storage items in their box and begin the inventory of storage items. Finally, place those items that will be kept where they belong after thoroughly cleaning the area.

Clean the area thoroughly before moving on to the next space. Each time a task is completed, like cleaning out that medicine cabinet, be sure to appreciate the success. It's crucial during this stage to monitor for distress. It's quite likely that any hoarder will experience challenging emotions as the decluttering proceeds. It's important to acknowledge those feelings and practice the CBT techniques for understanding and dealing with them. Having a support network on hand, particularly in the beginning of the declutter process and when clearing areas with numerous items of sentimental value. To be effective in support through this process, it's important that family and friends agree to a support schedule when they can be present to help as the individual proceeds through the declutter process. If the distress is severe, it is also acceptable to hire a professional cleaning service rather than decluttering personally. The point is to clear the clutter and treat the behavior that resulted in the accumulation in the first place.

It's common at the beginning of the process for them to feel overwhelmed by the amount of clutter. Don't let that become discouraging--remind them of that old adage about how to eat an elephant; one bite at a time. Visit the vision board to remember all the reasons for doing this work. The images of clean spaces and happy family events in a clutter-free environment serve as potent reminders for how life can be once the job is done. It's also important to call on the support network as needed. Hoarders will typically alternate between feelings of shame and hopelessness until real progress can be seen, and therefore, it's essential to have supportive family, friends, and even therapists at the ready to assist as necessary.

Finish the Area Before Moving On

Completely finish the work in the target area before moving on to another area. Again, it's important to consistently check in with the types of feelings and thoughts the person is experiencing as they proceed with decluttering. The negative feelings that arise should be thoughtfully considered and dealt with in accordance with the CBT techniques learned in therapy sessions. It's important to acknowledge positive feelings that arise, too. As areas are decluttered, it's common to feel a sense of satisfaction and accomplishment. These feelings should be savored and used for further motivation. And, the success of clearing a space should be celebrated, too. Remember that it's a step toward a healthier, happier life.

Review Accomplishments

Once an area has been cleaned, it should be checked off on the map. That engenders an enormous sense of satisfaction, which then provides motivation for continuing the process. It should become apparent through the decluttering process whether the individual is ready to handle the feelings they're experiencing during the process. If it is generating too much distress as they are attempting to throw things away, there are options to consider that can help. Family, friends, or a professional cleaning service can take over when the affected individual doesn't think they can continue. They should not interpret this as a failure; in fact, if they are having someone else continue the declutter process, that is still a success. Their main job is to manage the negative emotions and thoughts that are arising as they move on with decluttering their environment. That is the real work of treating this condition. A decluttered environment is merely a side effect of the healing process.

Chapter Summary

This chapter has presented information on how to proceed with the decluttering process. Specifically, information on the following topics has been covered:

- Selecting a high priority, low sentimental value area to begin;

- Selecting a small space within the area;
- Using the pomodoro technique and the two-minute rule;
- Staging the belongings;
- Decluttering by category;
- Finishing one area before moving on;
- Reviewing accomplishments and progress.

The next chapter will present information on how to handle deciding what to do with specific items.

I t's so easy for anyone to vacillate when trying to throw
something away. For a hoarder, it's even harder. That's
why it's important to know the individual's style or personality and to take it one individual object at a time, asking
some very specific questions about what to do with it.
Which box to put it in? Additionally, it's a good idea to set
strict guidelines that determine what to do depending on the
answers to those questions. The following tips can make the
process much easier.

Hoarder Personality

There are different kinds of hoarders, and it's helpful to
know the style of the clutter accumulation. That will be
helpful for identifying weak spots and clutter areas that

might be particularly problematic. Most people fall into one of three categories:

- **The Disorganized Collector**: This person buys duplicate items because they don't have an organized system for storing them, and then, when they need the item in a hurry, they can't find it. For that reason, they end up buying another one and the cycle starts anew.

- **The Saver**: This is the person who worries that they might need the object in the future. They save it, "just in case," but rarely actually need the item. They typically feel this way about every object regardless of the likelihood they actually will need it.

- **The Chronically Overwhelmed**: This individual feels constantly overwhelmed, and since they don't know where to begin with the declutter process, they consistently give up trying. As they accumulate objects, they may consider clearing them out, but the job feels like it's just too much, so they never do.

Be Prepared

Just like it's important to tackle one space at a time within the house, it's also important to make decisions about one object at a time. But, it's also critical to be prepared for those justifications that will undoubtedly arise. For example, many hoarders will use one of the following phrases in accordance with the personality types above. The phrases are: 1) "I have to go through those," common for the chronically over-whelmed, 2) "But, I need it," or a common saver variant, "Someone could use that," and 3) "I need a new one of these," common for the disorganized collector. It's helpful to actu-ally write these phrases (or whatever common justification phrase the individual uses) down. That way it's possible to anticipate the objections that might come up during the decluttering process.

When these phrases do come up, it's important to challenge them, so the person can see how they're a symptom of dysfunction. For example, "I have to go through those," can be challenged with, "That's what we're doing now." "I need it," or, "I need a new one of these," can be challenged with, "When was the last time you used it?" If the individual can't remember or knows it's been more than a year, then they really don't need it and they certainly don't need a new one.

Ask Questions

For each object, it's a good idea to ask some specific ques-tions about the item. They include the following:

- When was the last time this item was used?
- How important is this item?
- Does it have a specific use?
- If the answer is yes, what is that use and how often is it used?
- Did the person even remember that they had this item?
- Is this the only one of these the individual has?
- Is it so important that they would trade a sense of inner peace for it?

These questions will help you narrow down the decision about what to do with the item. For example, if it isn't something that gets used regularly or that the person even remembered having, then it probably isn't a necessary item to keep. That should help bolster the decision to throw it away or donate it to charity.

Set the Rules

It's a good idea to set specific guidelines regarding what to do depending on the answers to those questions. If these guidelines are set up and all parties agree to abide by them, then the decision is pretty much made depending on the answer to the questions. The questions and their answers can be set up like a flowchart. It could look something like this:

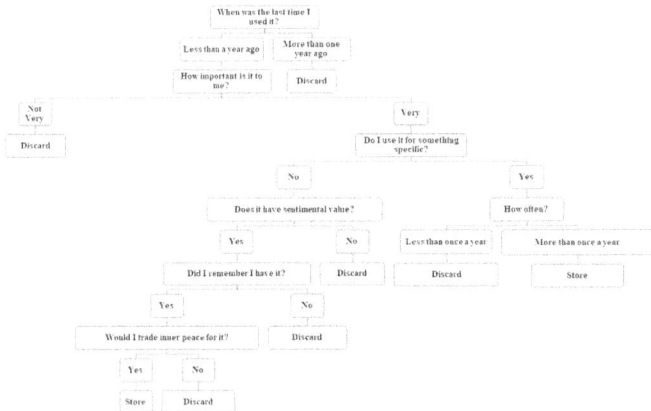

The answers to the questions on the flowchart leave little room for guesswork. The individual simply answers the questions and follows the flow. That will help eliminate any vacillation. If it's necessary to justify the decisions further, here are a few lines of logic that can help give the process more structure:

- If it hasn't been used in the last year, throw it away or donate it. Realistically speaking, if the object hasn't been used in that time, it's not something that is needed. There may be certain exceptions-- for example, it's possible that a jack for the car hasn't been used in the last year, but that kind of item should be kept--but, generally speaking, this is a good guideline.

- If it is not something that the person even

remembered having, then it can't have much sentimental value and it isn't very necessary--throw it away or donate it. Truly sentimental items are something that most people will display somewhere in the home and remember having.

- If it is something that is sentimental, it's important to consider if it's worth a sense of peace to keep. A memento from a vacation taken years ago might have sentimental value, but particularly if it hasn't been on display, it's probably not something worth sacrificing a sense of inner peace. Take a picture of it so that it can be stored digitally and throw it away or donate it.

To determine whether it is something that should or can be donated, it's helpful to ask a series of different questions:

- Is it in good condition?
- Is it in good enough condition to sell?
- Who is it designed for?
- Can it help someone else?

Most charities require that donations be in an acceptable condition, so if it isn't, then it goes into the trash box. It's possible to see how these questions form part of a system for determining what to do with the objects in your house. By setting down specific rules for what to do depending upon the answers to the questions, it removes the guesswork and leaves less room for indecision that can stall the process. This produces a specific plan of attack that streamlines the decluttering process. But, there's another rule that can help at this stage.

Use the OHIO Rule

The OHIO rule is used to help determine whether fears about letting go of an object are rational. OHIO stands for Only Handle It Once. Once the answer to the questions asked above yields a definitive action, and the object has been placed in the appropriate box, it should never be handled again. Of course, those items put in the "put away" box will be handled again when they are put away, but they should be put away as quickly as possible to ensure that there really is a place for them, and then, they can be enjoyed. For the rest of the boxes, leave those items alone, and move on to the next object.

This process can create anxiety in a hoarder. If the distress is significant, ask "What is the worst that can happen if the item is discarded? It's a good idea to allow them to express the fears they have about discarding the item. It's also important to validate those fears and show them compassion. No matter how unlikely the fears are, to an individual afflicted with hoarding disorder, they are real and imminent. By allowing them to express their fears, it is then possible to use CBT exercises to challenge those thoughts and emotions. That helps the individual to work through and challenge their own negative thoughts and fears, which then gives them the power and control over their response to decluttering. This makes them stronger as the process progresses.

It is important to constantly check in as the decluttering progresses. The individual should be encouraged to voice any and all distress so that it can be properly dealt with, and the internal healing can proceed. They should not be teased or judged for their feelings, because their feelings are valid. They need to voice them to be able to challenge them. And, they should know that should it get too stressful, it's always an option to call in help from family and friends or a CBT therapist. This will help keep the decluttering process on track, and more importantly, it will help them begin to get control over their worst fears.

Chapter Summary

This chapter has presented information on taking as much of the guesswork out of the decluttering process as possible. These specific topics were covered:

- Hoarder personality types: the disorganized collector, the saver, and the chronically overwhelmed;

- Preparation for typical justifications for each hoarder personality;
- Questions to ask about each object to determine which box it goes into;
- The OHIO rule;
- Constantly checking in with the affected person and how they are feeling.

The next chapter will present information for when the individual is unsure what to do with an object.

STEP 8: HAVE A SOLID STRATEGY FOR WHEN YOU'RE NOT SURE

For most hoarders, an excuse to delay a decision presents a risk for abandoning the declutter process. For that reason, it's best to have a plan of attack for those times when a person simply doesn't know what to do with an object. There will certainly be those types of objects, and thus, to avoid problems, a solid strategy will help. The following tips can help in such situations.

Create an "Unsure" Box

Creating an "unsure" box can be useful for those items they're not certain about. This is, however, a strategy that should be used with care. It's easy for a hoarder to want to put everything in that box. One strategy to avoid that is to only allow one unsure box for each space. That way, the box can't be used too frequently. It's also a good strategy to employ the flow chart for these types of items. If the object hasn't been used in more than a year or if the person didn't remember they had it, then that makes a strong argument for discarding or donating it.

If an unsure box is created, then it's important to also make a specific plan to revisit the box within a certain period of time, for example, six months. If, when the person later revisits that box, they have forgotten what was in it, or if the items in it were not needed in that period of time, again, it's a good argument for discarding the objects therein. If, on the other hand, the individual uses one or more of the objects in that box on a regular basis or finds a place in the home to display the item(s), then there is the answer.

It's also possible to get an answer more quickly. Maybe sleeping on it will help. Sometimes a period of unconsciousness can help with the decision-making process. Researchers have discovered that the brain is always working, even when a person is unconscious. During unconscious thought, the biases that a person feels during the waking state disappear. Thus, it's possible to weigh the importance of the components that are relevant to the decision more equally. That's why sleeping on it can be a helpful strategy. But, if this strategy is used, it's also important to resolve to make a decision in the morning.

The important thing, in this case, is to have a plan in place for dealing with those items. If the items are just put away in some box, the problem has not been resolved, and the box becomes another hoarded object. This is another situation where it's important to have a plan that all parties are willing to follow. It's fine to take more time to make a decision by thinking about it for six months, but it's important to follow through on it. If, in that time, there hasn't been a need for the object or it hasn't been missed, then that is essentially a decision made in and of itself.

Duplicates

Most hoarders have duplicates of many items, and so, this is another situation that requires preparation and a strategy for resolution. Often duplicates are of items that are common-place and easy to replace, for example, kitchen spatulas. Even so, hoarders are typically fearful of losing their things or being left without something they vitally need. For most hoarders, they struggle with the fear of decision-making and heightened emotional reactivity as part of the compulsive desire to keep the things they have, and when they are faced with discarding items, they respond with intense emotional reactions. That's part of why it's difficult to convince them of the irrational nature of their behavior. Even if they know on an intellectual level that they can easily replace that spatula, the problem is the intense emotions they may be feeling at the thought of discarding even a duplicate item.

This is why it is important to understand how to respond to those intense emotions when they arise. Because hoarders commonly fall into what are called "thinking traps," it can be useful to know how to deal with these. These thinking traps can goad anyone into more compulsive behavior as well as cause them to delay or abandon their efforts to heal their disorder. That's why it's worthwhile to examine some of the common thinking traps experienced by hoarders and methods for challenging those thoughts. The following table presents some common thinking traps and examples of thoughts experienced by people with hoarding disorder.

THINKING TRAPS: EXAMPLES

Thinking Traps	Examples
Fortune-telling: This is where the person will make often catastrophic predictions about what will happen as they move through the healing process. These kinds of thoughts are frequently triggered by the decluttering process.	*"I know I'll mess this up."* *"If I throw this away, I'll need it and won't be able to find another like it."* *"I will never be able to overcome my anxiety."*
Black-and-white thinking: This is where the person will think about a situation in terms of extremes. It's either all good or all bad, a success or a failure. While the declutter process is ongoing, if it's not been completed successfully, it's common for them to consider it an utter failure. This is true as well when they are faced with decision-making around items they're unsure about. They can easily view that as failure. In reality, there is a lot of gray area between the extremes.	*"Anything less than perfect is a failure."* *"Why do I still have problems with this? I should be cured by now."* *"I can't decide what to do with this item--I have totally failed to overcome this disorder!"*
Mind-reading: This frequently occurs as the person is certain they know what family, friends, and the therapist are thinking about them and their condition. Their sense of shame spurs this trap on, since they believe everyone is thinking the worst of them. The problem here is that most of the individual's friends and family just want to help.	*"Others think I'm stupid."* *"She or he doesn't like me."* *"They all think I'm crazy."*

Over-generalization:

The best way to recognize this is when the words "always" and "never" are used. This type of thinking fails to take all situations or events into account. Surely, everyone makes mistakes, but that doesn't mean they can't achieve their goals.

"I always make mistakes."

"I'll never be able to keep from hoarding."

"I'll never get this house decluttered."

Labeling:

This kind of behavior is reflective of the negative thoughts that are common to people affected by this disorder. CBT has specific ways to handle these types of thoughts, and that's one reason it is critical to the treatment of hoarding disorder. These negative thoughts undermine self-confidence and self-esteem. It's imperative for the individual to develop strategies for neutralizing negative thinking.

"I'm stupid."

"I'm crazy."

"I'm a loser."

Overestimation or Catastrophization:

"I will lose everything."

This kind of thinking is the result of the anxiety produced by the negative and obsessive thoughts. The person typically envisions the worst-case scenario, often resulting in an extreme or illogical conclusion.

"If I give up my stuff, I will never be able to have these things again."

"I will be unable to function."

A great way to help a hoarder overcome these kinds of thinking traps is to challenge those thoughts as they arise. It's important to clear this with the person's therapist, but by actively attempting to transform negative thoughts into positive ones, the individual will learn to deal with these kinds of thoughts as they arise. That's a skill that's useful for more than hoarding disorder. The following steps can be used to help reorient the thinking patterns.

- What was the situation that triggered the thoughts? Write this down and describe it in detail as it happened.

- What was the obsessive behavior that was triggered? Describe what the person was feeling the urge to do.

- Rate the strength of the feelings or urges on a scale of 0 to 10 with 0 being weak and 10 being very strong.

- Hoarder's interpretation of the feelings or urges-- describe this in detail.

- Balanced alternative interpretation--what is another more reasonable interpretation of the situation?

- Rate the individual's feelings about the balanced alternative interpretation on a scale of 0 to 10.

It might be helpful to illustrate these steps with an example. Considering the spatula example above, feelings of anxiety can easily be triggered when the person is prompted to consider discarding the duplicate items. When they recognize that they are feeling anxiety, it is a good exercise to have them stop and describe the situation that triggered those feelings. They might say something like, "As I was cleaning out my kitchen utensils, I encountered duplicate spatulas. I immediately began to feel anxiety upon thinking about discarding the duplicates. I had an immediate, strong urge to hide the items rather than discard them so that I would have them should I need them. I kept thinking that I might run out of spatulas and be unable to cook my food. The feeling was very strong. I would rate it an 8 out of 10. It caused me to freeze, and I found I could not continue the declutter process at that moment. My heart rate increased as did my breathing. That caused me to feel shame, because I'm not better yet. I thought I was getting better, but I still have such anxiety over something as stupid as a spatula."

Now, challenge those thoughts with these questions:

- Am I falling into a thinking trap, e.g. *catastrophizing* or *overestimating danger?*
- What is the evidence that what I'm thinking is true? What is the evidence that what I'm thinking is not true?
- Am I confusing a thought with a fact?
- What would I tell my best friend if he or she had the same thought?
- What would a friend tell me about this thought?
- Am I 100% sure that _____ will happen?
- Has it happened before, and if so, how many times?
- Is _____ so important that my future depends on it?
- What is the worst thing that could happen?

- If it did happen, what would I do to cope with it, what strategies am I learning that could help me to handle it?
- Am I basing my judgment of this situation on my feelings or on facts?
- Am I confusing "possibility" with "certainty"? It may be possible, but is it likely?

With these questions answered, it's now important for the person to devise a balanced alternative interpretation of the situation. The first thing to do is identify the thinking trap. There are several kinds here--there are elements of black and white thinking, over-generalization, and fortune-telling. Identifying the specific thinking trap can help with the reorientation of the thoughts and feelings the individual is experiencing. So, what would be a balanced alternative interpretation? It could look something like this: "It's so easy to accumulate numerous items like these spatulas. They are inexpensive and easy to find. My feelings of anxiety about these duplicates are understandable given my disorder, but I'm making progress by working to declutter my home. I understand that this is a process and it takes time. I resolve to be patient and compassionate with myself. Discarding duplicates is part of that process, and the urges the thought of that triggered are merely side effects of the healing process. I know that should I require another spatula for any reason, I can easily acquire one, and even if my current spatula broke while I was using it, I could still use other utensils to finish cooking my food. The anxiety that was triggered initially is completely understandable given the decluttering process I am undertaking. I will continue to declutter my environment, because I know I am strong enough to take control over my obsessive urges. I love a challenge and I can do this!"

The balanced alternative interpretation is compassionate and recognizes the difficulty faced by the individual when undertaking decluttering procedures. It's important for them to recognize the feelings that arise as they move through the process. That is part of the healing they are seeking. Helping them to see the alternative thinking processes that are available will help alleviate their stress, and it will also train their brain to think more positively. Like any other habit, negative or positive thinking patterns create and strengthen neural pathways in the brain, which makes it easier for the brain to go down the same route the next time. For most hoarders, the negative thinking pathways have been strengthened over time. But, it's possible to retrain the brain to use strong positive thinking neural pathways instead. To do that requires vigilance with one's thoughts and feelings, and it requires taking the time consistently to replace negative thoughts with positive ones (Firestone, 2018; Oppong, 2018).

By dealing with negative feelings that arise during the decluttering process, it will also help to appreciate the strategies developed to deal with situations like duplicates and items the person is unsure about. That will help to keep the process going and everyone motivated.

Chapter Summary

This chapter has presented information on dealing with items an individual is uncertain about and duplicate items. Specifically, the following topics were covered:

- The "unsure" box and how to handle it;
- Why sleeping on it can help with the decision-making process;
- Putting the unsure box away for six months and revisiting those items at that time;
- How to deal with duplicate items;
- How duplicate items and uncertainty can cause a person to fall into thinking traps;
- The different kinds of thinking traps;
- How to challenge the validity of thinking traps and negative thinking.

The next chapter will present information on scaling down collections.

STEP 9: SCALE DOWN YOUR COLLECTIONS

L arge collections of items can cause significant clutter, and often, they are things that don't really add to a person's quality of life. Still, people often spend many years collecting items in which they are particularly interested. Getting rid of those collections can be very distressing, so an alternate strategy is to scale them down instead. There are a number of ways to downsize any type of collection or memorabilia. It is important to understand that collections don't refer to duplicate items; rather, these are the kinds of things, like Hummel figurines, that form part of a collection. It also includes family memorabilia. While there are several reasons to keep these, they can add up to significant clutter, and that means it is necessary to develop a strategy for dealing with them. The strategy depends in part on the items being collected. The following strategies can be helpful.

Keep Some Items

Keep a few items from each collection instead of the whole collection. Pick out some of the more valuable or rare items in the collection. If numerous parts are kept in the home, keep them together so that they aren't scattered in different areas of the home. If the collection really is something of value to the person, then they should wish to display it. If not, it might be wise to consider if it is worth keeping at all. If the entire collection is something valuable, but it can't all be displayed, then one option is to display the more interesting or valuable items and store the rest. As with anything else that is stored, it's important to have an inventory on the box so that the items can be located easily. This will reduce the clutter, but make it easy to find the remaining items whenever necessary.

Consider Alternative Storage Strategies

Keeping part of the collection can help to reduce the anxiety generated by thinking about getting rid of it, but it's also important to spend some time thinking about whether it really adds value to life. If the collection involves something like magazines, cards, or pictures, the question is whether these will ever be used. Furthermore, are they being stored properly? If it is something that the individual really wants to keep, it might be worthwhile to explore alternative storage strategies. Pictures or cards could be put into a scrapbook for storage. That would help provide them with proper storage where they could be protected from deterioration due to environmental exposure. This would also provide them with a way to easily access the collection and show it to family and friends. For other types of items, like magazines, it might be worthwhile to consider the value of keeping these kinds of items. For this kind of thing, it might be better to keep some of the collection--the most notable or important issues, for example--and donate the remainder to a library where they can properly curate the collection. It might even be possible that they will make a note of the name of the individual who donated the collection.

Family Memorabilia

Collections also include family memorabilia, and that can be particularly difficult to downsize because of the attached sentimental value. These kinds of materials are also often tied to family histories and a sense of heritage. Many hoarders attach a sense of responsibility in overseeing the family heritage. That can make these kinds of things particularly difficult to deal with during the decluttering process. So, how can these kinds of items be dealt with when decluttering? It can be helpful to answer the following questions:

- **Do I love this and/or will I use this in my home?** Though the memorabilia that many people inherit from their family may be interesting, the items are often not something that they will really use in their home. They frequently start out keeping them because of feelings of obligation, but the reality is that unless the item is something that is being used, why store it simply for reasons of family history? The family history can be documented in other ways. For example, it's possible to photograph the item and describe what is known about its history and the importance to the family--for example, when was it acquired, is there a date associated with it, or is there a particular relative who originally bought or made it. Documenting that kind of information adds value to the item. Then, if it is not something being used, it can be donated or sold along with its provenance or history. Antique dealers will want that kind of information. And, the person still has the information about the item and its place in their family history.

- **Is this item really valuable to the family history?** There are a number of things that people acquire over the course of their lifetime. No one knows that better than a hoarder, but many of those items are not particularly significant in the life of the owner. Much of what a person might inherit will be nothing more than useless items that have little value to their family history. These might include things like paperwork that has no value or items that, though old, were and are still commonplace, meaning they will have little value as antiques. Those kinds of things can easily be discarded.

- **Is this something my children will want someday?** There are certain things that children may eventually appreciate having as they grow older. War medals, family artwork, or items made by family members are possible examples. These are the kinds of things that might be worth storing to give to children someday. But, it's also true that many things won't hold the same sentimental value for the children as they might for older generations. Grandma's china might be important to her daughter, but her granddaughter might find it outdated. Thus, those things that are unlikely to hold meaning for the younger generations can be discarded.

- **Are the items in good condition?** This is an important consideration for whether to keep them or discard them. Old books, photographs, and other memorabilia might have real value, but if they aren't in good condition, that can negatively impact any resale value, and if it is not possible to properly curate them to prevent further deterioration, there is no reason to keep them. It might be worthwhile to find someone who can try to salvage those kinds of items and either donate or sell them to that person.

- **Is there something unique about the item?** Another consideration when deciding whether to keep or discard an item is if it is, in some way, unique. Antiques that have real value are usually rare. Items that were mass-produced or for which there are numerous examples will have less value than those items that are unique. If there is a question, it might be worthwhile to take the item to an expert who can help to evaluate its value. If it has no value, then it might be better to discard it.

- **If I do not want to display the item, do I have space to store it properly?** This is another important consideration. If the item will not be on display, is it possible to store it properly so that it doesn't deteriorate? If this is the decision, it's also wise to ask what purpose storing it will serve. Why keep something that won't be used or displayed? If the individual feels significant distress at making a decision regarding the item, perhaps for reasons of sentimental value, this might be an option, but like the "unsure" box, it is a good idea to revisit this decision in six months.

Letting go can be a difficult process, but it doesn't represent a loss, it represents a new beginning. It's helpful to remember the reasons for decluttering, and to focus on the new, positive feelings that will result from a decluttered environment. If the person is experiencing significant stress over this process, it might be time to revisit the vision board for reminders of just why this is a good process and all of the positive things to come.

Chapter Summary

This chapter has presented information on scaling down collections. Specifically, the following topics were covered:

- How collections differ from duplicate items;
- Strategies for dealing with collections;
- Keep some of the collection;
- Alternative storage strategies;
- How to deal with family memorabilia.

The next chapter will present information on how to be ruthless in the decluttering process.

STEP 10: BE RUTHLESS AND START AGAIN

W hen decluttering a house, it can be necessary to be absolutely ruthless. Having a plan in place to deal with the clutter will help with this. It can be difficult to do, but it's easier if it is done with much thought. That can be done for the kinds of things that are obviously trash. It's so easy to hoard household items, for example; things like beauty products, cleaning products, or stationery. The easiest strategy for trying to declutter their house is to just throw these kinds of items away. If necessary, make the decision to buy one replacement of every essential, but get rid of the old items. These are the half-filled shampoo bottles, the dozens of travel-sized soaps, and the hotel body lotions collected over numerous vacations.

Throw Them Out

As was mentioned, it's best to stage the items in a space that's being cleaned. For example, pull everything out of the cabinets under the bathroom sink, and divide the materials into piles by types. For example, put all of the cleaning supplies in one pile, things like toilet paper in another, and body lotion in yet another. With this strategy items that are trash will become readily apparent. Throw those things out right away without even thinking about it. Unless the item is something that is currently being used, it's best to get rid of it. That makes it easier to clean quickly, which results in a great sense of satisfaction. It also has the added benefit of helping to retrain the brain with positive feelings of a job well done. Remember that these kinds of items can be easily replaced, and so, don't allow anxiety about throwing them away to creep in and disrupt the flow of the work.

This is a good strategy for all items that don't hold sentimental value. It's the "fresh start" approach and it can help to clean things very quickly and easily. It is necessary, however, to be absolutely ruthless and rigidly consistent. In fact, it's best to act before there is even time to think about it--just scoop up all of those half-filled bottles into a trash bag, each and every one. Remember, this is an opportunity for a fresh start. By acting quickly and decisively, it will eliminate any question about what to do with the items. They're out before there's even a question about it. And, remember the OHIO rule. Once they're in the trash, they shouldn't be handled again.

It's common as part of this direct, abrupt activity to have some doubts, but these tips can help to alleviate any stress that arises as part of this process.

- **The 80/20 rule**: This rule was originally developed in relation to clothing. It states that a person generally only wears approximately 20 percent of the clothing they own an astonishing 80 percent of the time. While it was developed for clothing, it also works for other items. For example, most people tend to listen to 20 percent of their music collection 80 percent of the time. They play 20 percent of their video game collection 80 percent of the time, and so on. The goal for decluttering is to get rid of the things that go unused 80 percent of the time.
- **Don't worry about sunk costs**: Economists define sunk costs as those costs that have already been incurred and cannot be recovered. Except for rare items that increase in value over time, the majority of things in anyone's house can be thought of as sunk costs. The money it took to purchase them cannot be recouped. For that reason, it is better to think about the value added by discarding

the item as part of the decluttering process rather than the money it cost to purchase it. That money is already gone and cannot be retrieved. Understanding the concept of sunk costs can help for making more rational decisions about the objects in the house.

- **If it's broken, don't fix it**: It's not uncommon to discover long-forgotten treasures as part of the decluttering process. But, if the item doesn't work, it won't help to keep it stored in the house for another moment, day, week, or month. Get rid of it. It's a sunk cost and it doesn't work. The decision is really an easy one, it's out.

- **Track the items that get used**: A clever way to do this during the preparation for decluttering is to put an item back where it lives to face the opposite direction of the other items around it. For example, if it's an item of clothing, hang it in the opposite direction of the other clothing items in the closet or put it back in the drawer upside down in comparison to the other clothes. This is an easy way to see what is getting used and what isn't. When it comes time to declutter, it's easier to simply pull out those items that are not being used and discard them without thinking about it. Again, be ruthless.

- **Clear off flat surfaces**: Flat surfaces are easy places to pile things up, and they're a good place to start with decluttering. Be ruthless in throwing out the junk mail that gets stashed on the kitchen countertop, put away the pens used for making the grocery list in a drawer, and commit to keeping only a few essential, small appliances on those countertops. If there are items that never get used, consider donating them or throwing them out. Again, if it's something that hasn't been used in over a year, it's not important and can be discarded.

- **Store like with like**: Organize the storage for the items that will be kept so that like items are stored together. This makes it much easier to find them when they are needed, and it keeps everything organized nicely. This will not only help declutter the home, it will also reduce the stress of not being able to find something when it's needed.

- **Ask if an item will be used**: If there is something that can be used, that does not mean it is something that will be used. Be honest about the items that will be used, and donate, sell, or throw out those items that won't get used, no matter how interesting or useful they might be. If they won't be used, they're just taking up space.

- **More is not better**: It's not necessary to have

two microwave ovens, four spatulas, or three blow dryers. It's easy to think that there's a back up if one breaks, but the reality is that most of these items are easily replaced if that happens. There's no reason to keep duplicate items. Be ruthless and get rid of them.

- **Avoid overthinking**: This is the benefit of acting ruthlessly and quickly, it's possible to avoid overthinking. If not, it's easy to get into a cycle of going through a complicated decision-making process. This can be avoided by having a strict policy regarding categorizing items and acting on the answers to the questions discussed in earlier chapters.

- **Don't judge**: As part of this process, problems will crop up and it's not uncommon for hoarders to judge themselves as inadequate. They've made the decision to declutter and seek treatment, but it can seem like a very slow process. And, when mistakes happen, they often feel discouraged. The job doesn't have to be perfect; it's okay to make mistakes, so don't judge too harshly. Treatment for hoarding disorder can be a long process and there may be setbacks. The important thing is to stay on track.

- **Have courage**: Beating this disorder can be scary. The person affected will confront some very uncomfortable feelings and thoughts during the decluttering process, and it takes courage to face those fears. The very fact that they have chosen to work through this process is a testament to their strength. But, it takes courage to face those fears and risk making a wrong decision.

- **Be patient**: Recovering from a hoarding disorder is a process. It will take time, so focus on those small victories, take time to celebrate the progress, and keep going.

- **Keep on trucking**: It's easy to become overwhelmed by the decluttering process, but it's vital to keep going. Don't stop, even for a day. Maybe it's not possible to do more than just five minutes of decluttering a day, but that's good enough. It keeps the ball rolling so that the process is not stalled.

- **Be strict**: Make a commitment to the process by setting rules. For example, no TV until after the day's decluttering has been accomplished. This will help establish a reward for the day's efforts, and that can help in the process of retraining the brain, which is always looking for a reward.

- **Ask for help when it's needed**: There is never any shame in admitting that you require help. It's important to remember that it takes courage to ask someone for help. That might be friends or family members who are part of a support network or it could be a therapist. It makes no difference--reach out when necessary. Even if it just helps to have someone in the home as the decluttering process is proceeding, ask for help. Your support network is there for just this reason.

When setbacks are encountered, start the process over again. Don't let a relapse stop you from continuing with the healing process. Setbacks are inevitable when dealing with a challenging disorder such as this, but they don't mean that the process has failed. It's just a setback. Like every other part of the decluttering process, develop a strategy for dealing with setbacks. That may require calling the therapist or other members of the support network, but it also means reflecting on the reasons for the setback. It can help to keep a journal of the emotions triggered during the declutter process and any setbacks encountered along the way. Maintaining a journal can reveal patterns for the problems encountered during decluttering. For example, it might reveal the more common or powerful triggers, the patterns of thoughts and emotions that cause the greatest problems, and those emotions that come to the surface when significant progress is made.

Keeping a journal can also be a useful way to challenge negative thoughts and emotions. It can be used to document those thought traps and challenge their rationality. It can also help the person gain a deeper understanding of the underlying psychological problems that helped create the problem in the first place. This is a useful and illuminating strategy that helps with both the decluttering process and in maintaining a decluttered environment. And, it provides a non-judgemental outlet for the thoughts and emotions that so frequently grip a hoarder while attempting to declutter. This is where they can speak freely about the ideas that come to mind, the fears that threaten to derail their progress, and the hopes that keep them going. This is an area where a ruthless and strict attitude is necessary too. Be ruthless about recording those thoughts and emotions that arise each and every day. That's a good habit to develop.

Chapter Summary

This chapter has presented information on being ruthless during the declutter process. Specifically, the following topics were covered:

- Being ruthless in the process of discarding duplicate items;
- Tips for alleviating stress as part of the declutter process;

- The 80/20 rule and its broad application;
- If it's broken, get rid of it;
- Be patient and compassionate with yourself;
- Ask for help when needed;
- Respect the process.

The next chapter will present information on alternative ways to maintain cherished memories without adding to the clutter.

STEP 11: FIND AN ALTERNATIVE WAY TO KEEP MEMORIES

One of the biggest problems for hoarders are items of sentimental value. It's hard for anyone to let go of those, but it's also easy to attach sentimental value to an item as a justification for keeping it. That's why it's important to address these items in some very special ways. There are a few strategies that can help with these kinds of items.

Why is the Item Important?

Before undertaking this process, it is important to ascertain what the item really means to the individual. A few directed questions can help to understand the sentimental value it holds.

- Where did this item come from?
- What does it mean to the individual?

- Why exactly are they sentimental about it? Usually, it's not the object per se, but it's attachment to a particular person or event that gives it a sentimental value.
- Is this something that can be displayed in the home rather than stored?
- Is the item in good condition? If not, it's better to photograph it and discard the object.

Process Feelings of Attachment

It's also a good idea when processing sentimental items to process the feelings that they represent. It's important for people affected with hoarding disorder to understand that the object is not the feeling or the memory. Those are something that resides within each person. The object simply evokes the memory. Thus, it is possible to take a picture of the item and use that to honor those special people and events in each person's life.

Discarding items of sentimental value will take some time. It is difficult to let them go, and there certainly may be some objects the person will keep--perhaps the most favorite items or those in the best condition. It may take several sessions of decluttering to get through these kinds of items. That's okay, because it's important to process those feelings.

Get Rid of Any Guilt

Sometimes people hold on to items not because they are sentimental about them, but because they feel guilty. They might feel bad about a relationship with the person who is attached to the item, and they keep the item because they feel guilty about not repairing the relationships. Unfortunately, guilt is a useless emotion. It won't fix any relationship or undo any action taken in the past, and neither will keeping the item to which the sentimental value is attached. Guilt is a particularly unhelpful emotion that needs to be processed and let go of. Sometimes just recognizing the real reason behind the sentimentality can be enough to let go of the object, but other times it may be necessary to process the feelings in a different way. Here are a few tips:

- **Understand the feeling**: Before anything can be done about feelings of guilt, it is imperative to first understand the root cause. By identifying specifically what the individual feels guilty about, it will then be possible to move on from the feeling.

- **Talk about it**: As with almost any other feeling, it's important to talk it out with a trusted friend, loved one, or professional. They have a much less biased perspective on the situation and can offer the kind of support to help eliminate guilty feelings.

- **Practice self-compassion**: One way to do this

is to imagine that it is a good friend who has this problem. It's helpful to think about the advice that a person would give to their best friend who came to them with this problem. Most people would be compassionate with their best friend, and if that's the case, why not be compassionate with themselves? This is not simply excusing bad behavior, but it is understanding the context in which the behavior occurs. The when and the why of the situation are important to understanding any reaction. By understanding those elements of the behavior, it is then also possible to have compassion for the response, even if it was inappropriate. Once there is self-compassion, it is possible to practice self-forgiveness, and that allows someone to make amends for their past actions. If they haven't forgiven themselves for their behavior, making amends will be more difficult.

- **Make amends**: Rather than living a lifetime with the guilt of past actions, why not simply make amends? It's not possible to undo the action and it may not be possible to undo the consequences that ensued, but it is minimally possible to express remorse and ask forgiveness.

- **Ask a Pro**: If the feelings of guilt are too difficult

to overcome, it's helpful to discuss them with a professional therapist. They can help the individual get to the root of their guilty feelings and move on from this distinctly unhelpful emotion.

Gifts Should Not Be Burdens

Many people hold onto items because they think the person will expect to see them when they visit. That may or may not be true, but even if it is, it's unfair for a gift-giver to have that expectation. It is, after all, a gift, which means it is the recipient's prerogative to do with it as they see fit. This can become a boundary-setting issue that might need to be addressed. If the gift giver were to ask about the gift, the recipient should be able to tell them that, though they appreciate the giver's thoughtfulness, the item just wasn't a fit for the home, and thus, it was given to someone who would truly appreciate it. It's important here to understand that no one controls another person's feelings, and if the giver is offended, they should also properly process their feelings to fully understand why. But, whether they do that or not isn't something under the control of the recipient.

Virtual Memories

One great way to maintain the sentimental value of an item without actually keeping the item is to create a digital filing system. This is where you take photographs of your sentimental items. By doing this, you can keep the memories the item represents without actually keeping the item itself. This is particularly helpful for things like childhood artwork, memorabilia, magazine articles, and any other kind of paper item. It's also great for physical photographs, letters, documents, and greeting cards.

A good way to start is by organizing a filing system on whatever form of Cloud storage is available--Dropbox, Google Drive, iCloud, Evernote, etc.. In these systems, it is possible to create folders for things like childhood memories, projects, arts and crafts, letters, important documents, etc.. Once that has been accomplished, it's a simple matter of taking photographs of the items. It might be a good idea, depending on the item to take a photograph of each side. Once the photographs have been taken, they should be uploaded to the cloud storage, and then the physical item can be discarded.

Uploading these items to their digital file immediately can help ease your anxiety around getting rid of the physical item. And, this can also be done for objects like ornaments or jewelry that you don't need anymore, but they remind you of someone special or a special event. The great thing about this technique is that it allows you to access your memories more easily than if you had to sift through piles of stuff in your house or even locate the item in a box some-

where. Additionally, knowing that you can see your trea-
sured memories anytime you like can help ease your anxiety
about discarding the item.

Donate Significant Objects

Another good idea for preserving objects that the individual
feels deserve special respect is to donate the item. If it is an
antique, it might be possible to donate it to an archive or
local history museum. This is a great way to declutter
without discarding the item, but the item should be
researched in order to determine if it has value and will be
accepted by the organization.

Pass It On

Again, for those objects which the individual feels have
value, but which they don't wish to keep, a good option is to
pass them on. Even though one person might consider the
items trash, another family relative might find them valuable. Consult other family members to see if anyone would
like to have the object or objects in question.

Repurpose It

For those items which are in poor condition or unfit for
sale, it's always possible to repurpose the item into something that can be used. For example, the stone from a
grandparent's ring can be reset in a band that's more

modern. A board from an antique dresser can be turned into a floating shelf. That allows the person to keep part of the item for its sentimental value while getting rid of the remainder.

Keep Part of a Collection

Decluttering a collection with sentimental value can be particularly difficult. But, it is possible to keep part of the collection and let the rest go. For example, keep one or two items that are representative of the collection, person, or era and that will make it easier to let the remainder go.

Give It a New Home

Some items may hold a particular sentimental value, such that the individual has difficulty deciding between storing it forever and discarding it. For these kinds of objects, there may be another option. Perhaps, there's a friend who would love to have the item or someone else who really needs it. That way, the individual can be assured the item is going to a good home.

Make a Scrapbook

Making a scrapbook is simple and requires very little in the way of supplies; it only requires a simple, unlined notebook and a glue stick. And, a scrapbook makes a good place to store documents or pictures that have sentimental value or are an important part of the individual's life. The items can be preserved without taking up too much space.

These are great tips for dealing with items of sentimental value or those memories that are particularly important to preserve. Memorabilia can be particularly difficult for individuals suffering from hoarding disorder to organize, store, or discard. It's tempting to want to keep everything that is part of an individual's life, but it is possible to keep the memories without keeping the items themselves. The most important part of the decluttering process, particularly when dealing with these kinds of items, is to process the feelings that will undoubtedly arise during this part of the process. Individuals with hoarding disorder should be encouraged to voice their feelings and helped as they attempt to process them. Once they have mastered that skill, the decluttering process will become much easier.

Chapter Summary

This chapter has presented information on how to deal with decluttering memorabilia and items of sentimental value. Specifically, the following topics were covered:

- Determining why the item is important;
- Processing any feelings that arise as part of the decluttering process;

- Getting rid of any guilt associated with a perceived need to retain objects;
- Preventing gifts from becoming burdens;
- Various options for dealing with memorabilia.

The next chapter will present information on organizing, labeling, and storing those items that will be kept.

STEP 12: CHANNEL YOUR NEED FOR CONTROL INTO LABELING AND ORGANIZING

Most hoarders have a compulsive need to control their environment; that's part of the hoarding disorder. But, the energy that's behind that can be put to a more useful purpose, like organizing the declutter plan and categorizing and organizing those items which will be kept. Part of the problem with clutter is the impact it has on an individual's physical and mental health. Aside from the environmental hazards created by clutter, such as dust, mold, and fire hazards, there are other effects on an individual's physical and mental health. Clutter affects food choices which can contribute to obesity. It also affects interpersonal relationships, and it contributes to stress and depression.

Benefits of Organization

There are a number of benefits to decluttering and getting organized. Organization can help individuals sleep better, it can reduce stress, improve relationships, and allow a person to focus on other areas of their life in order to free up time and energy for improvements in those areas. Organization can also reduce depression and anxiety, result in better food choices, and help an individual lose weight. Finally, organization can help an individual be more productive.

How to Get Organized

Once the individual's environment is decluttered, it's time to organize those items that will be kept and stored in the home. This is an important part of the process since the individual will be living with those items for the foreseeable future. As with the decluttering process, planning is key. It's essential to make sure there is a place for everything that will be kept. Then, it will be important to get the necessary supplies. Make sure that everything is ready prior to proceeding so that there is no reason to delay. It's also a good idea to proceed systematically as was done during the decluttering process. Use the map again and proceed through each area on the map. The plan is to clean each area well and put the items that belong in that space away. To do that, it will require some supplies, including containers and container organizers. The following tips should help with the process.

Tips for Getting and Staying Organized

Here are some tips to get the organization process going and to make it much easier to do:

- **Clean**: Before putting anything away, clean the areas where the items will go. It's important to make sure everything is clean to begin.
- **Buy storage containers**: It's important to wait until this point to buy the storage containers since they will be a source of temptation during the decluttering process.
- **Find a home**: For the items to keep, find a place for them. Be sure to find a place for every object. They should be located in appropriate rooms of the house, and in appropriate spaces within the room. If there's any indecision as to where an object should go, don't just put it on an open surface. That makes it too easy to slip back into hoarding behaviors. Instead, create an unsure container, and when everything else is finished, then go back and make a decision about where to put the items in that box.
- **Categorize Containers**: Each container in a room where items will be stored should be

categorized by the type of item they will contain. For example, silverware drawer, spare batteries drawer, etc. can all be categories for drawers. That makes it easy to decide what goes in that drawer, cupboard, or box. Labeling each container will provide an even greater sense of control over the individual's environment.

- **Use open containers**: Use open containers to initially organize items, and then place those open containers inside the appropriately labeled drawer, box, or cupboard. By using this kind of rigid system, it will help with resisting the urge to sink back into disorganized hoarding behavior patterns. It will also help when putting things away. It's easy to toss items into an open container.

- **Open spaces**: Don't clutter up open spaces like tabletops. To avoid this, it can help to place something like flowers on the table. That will help prevent using the open space as a dumping ground for other objects.

- **No stacking**: Don't stack objects on top of one another. It can be tempting to do just that, but that's a great way to create clutter. Make sure that everything has its own space without having to be set on top of something else.

- **Create spaces that have limits**: This will help to prevent acquiring excess items in any one category. For example, if one drawer is for utensils, then if that drawer is filled and there are still more utensils, that indicates there's more decluttering work to do. And, over time, as that drawer gets full, it will serve as an indicator that it's time to address the problem again before it gets out of hand.

- **Every container should have container organizers**: Within each container used for organization, it's essential to include container organizers. Rather than simply throwing items into a drawer, for example, use container organizers to separate the areas within the drawer for use in storing specific items. Rubber bands can go in one area and batteries in another. In this way, even the all-purpose drawer can be organized properly.

- **Eliminate clutter hot spots**: There are places in every home that seem to be clutter magnets. These include places like an entryway table, kitchen counters, and the dining room table. Clear these areas of clutter accumulation each night before going to bed. Making it part of the daily routine can help prevent clutter accumulation. It can also help to put something on tables, like a flower arrangement, in order to take up the space so that there is less available for clutter.

- **Store a discard bag in the closet**: Use this bag for those clothes that no longer fit, are stained or out of style, or that just seem unflattering. Everyone has likely experienced buying clothing that seemed to look good in the store, but when they get it home, it suddenly seems less attractive. This bag is for those kinds of clothes. When the bag is full, it's time to make a donation to the thrift store.

- **Arrange items according to how frequently they're used**: Items that are used daily should be kept in plain sight or at eye level. Things used less frequently can be stored on higher shelving, and those things rarely used can be stored in an attic or storage shed. This will make it easier to find things that are used often, and it will also be easier to locate those things not used as frequently.

- **Be selective about what is brought into the home**: Be selective about what is brought into the home now that it's clean and organized. Consider what is needed, and for those things that are desirable, be sure they fit, there's space to store the item(s), and/or there are no unnecessary duplicates. It's also a good idea to use the one item in, one item out rule. If something is brought into the home, something should be taken out. That will help prevent unnecessary clutter buildup.

- **Set limits**: For those items like memorabilia or knick-knacks, assign them a limited area for storage. If that area gets full, that indicates there's no more room. Be strict about not bringing any more items in that category if the storage space is full.

- **Set a deadline**: For any unfinished storage projects, set a deadline. For example, by agreeing to host a family dinner, that will create a deadline for hanging those family photos in the living room. By making plans that will require the completion of the project, that will provide motivation to get it done.

- **Put things away**: Putting things away is a habit like any other, but it's a necessary one to develop in order to avoid accumulating more clutter. If things are not returned to their proper location, it will be easy to accumulate significant amounts of clutter quickly. By putting things away after using them, it will prevent the clutter accumulation and take much less time to keep things clean. It will also make it much easier to find things when necessary.

- **Appraise the system**: Once a space has been

decluttered and organized, take a look around to see if it looks clean. If it still looks messy, then there is more organization to be done. And, it can also indicate that improvements to the organizational system are necessary.

- **Be objective**: Look around the home in the same way a visitor would in order to assess any areas of clutter that can easily be overlooked. Walk through the home with fresh eyes and look for any areas of clutter build up. It can help to snap a picture of the room too. It can be easier to see clutter in a photograph that is easily overlooked when looking at the area.

By organizing and labeling spaces in your home, you'll regain a sense of control that your hoarding behavior had given you previously. Additionally, organizing helps your mental health by reducing anxiety and depression. The decluttering process will have been difficult, and you may find you have an increased anxiety level, but you can reduce that anxiety by taking back the control through organizing and labeling.

Chapter Summary

This chapter presented information on organizing belongings following the decluttering process. Specifically, the following topics were covered:

- The benefits of organization;
- How to get organized;
- Tips for getting and staying organized.

The next chapter will present information on a final, thorough cleaning.

STEP 13: A FINAL CLEAN

The final step in the decluttering process is to clean the whole area. Once everything is organized and put in its final place, cleaning will be an easier process. Each section will have been cleaned during the decluttering process, and thus, this part will not be as difficult as it would have been if it had been done sooner. At this point, deep cleaning will be the final step.

After years of hoarding, a deep clean will make sure the home is sanitary and a comfortable place to live. Here are a few suggestions for approaching a deep clean:

- Consider hiring a professional service, particularly for areas with heavy grime or in the event the task seems too daunting.
- If there are areas that need repair work as you're

cleaning, fix these as they are encountered or hire a handyman to the job. This is important to ensure that the space is safe and in good working order. That will also make it easier to resist returning to those old hoarding ways.

- Once the home is clean, remove any trash bags and take pictures of the home in its pristine condition. That will be a good reminder for all the reasons to undertake this process in the first place. It will also serve as motivation to stick to those future goals. The photos will also provide an easy reference for how nice the home looks when it is uncluttered and well-organized.

When undertaking the deep cleaning process, there are a number of things to consider. The first is that deep cleaning, like the decluttering and organizational processes, should be undertaken in a systematic manner. It's important to acquire all of the necessary supplies first, and then, proceed through the home in a systematic manner. The following information presents suggestions for how to proceed.

Supplies

As with any other part of this process, it's vital to have the proper supplies before getting started. At a minimum the following items will be required for a thorough cleaning:

- Disposable rags, scrub pads, or towels that can be thrown way when the job is complete;
- Two buckets--one for clean water and the other for dirty water;
- Degreaser, dish soap, and disinfectant spray--be sure to get enough of these for the entire job;
- Rubber gloves;
- An abrasive scrub pad;
- A spray bottle with a 1:1 vinegar to water solution. Vinegar is a great cleaner;
- A scrub brush and/or an old toothbrush;
- Cleaning products like glass cleaner, wood polish, etc.

For each of these items, be sure to get enough to finish the entire job. Obtaining the supplies prior to cleaning will be easier than having to stop and buy more supplies. Those kinds of delays can derail the motivation to keep going.

Deep Cleaning Process

As with the other parts of the decluttering process, this goes more smoothly if it is done in a systematic manner. Here are some suggestions for some of the more challenging areas of the home.

Deep Cleaning the Kitchen

Oven and Stovetop: The oven might have a self-cleaning feature, but these vary in how effective they are, and it's important to remove all materials that might be a fire hazard before employing the self-cleaner. Use the abrasive scrub pad and degreaser to remove baked-on food. An alternative to this is to make a vinegar and baking soda paste and let it sit on the food spills in the oven for about an hour before cleaning it off. Clean the baked-on food off the oven surface and then clean the wire racks.

Once the oven is complete, clean the stovetop by removing the pot grates and soaking them in hot, soapy water. If the oven is electric, it is also possible to remove/unplug the coils in order to facilitate the cleaning process. If the oven or cooktop has a slide-out tray beneath the burners, be sure to remove and clean those. Scrub all of the surfaces, including the control knobs, with a soapy sponge and a wet rag soaked in clean water. Be sure to also clean the hood fan and hood fan filter.

Microwave: Use a lemon and vinegar mix to loosen food splatters. Then, clean the inside with a soapy sponge and wet rag. Remove the plate platform and clean that using dish soap and water. Glass cleaner can be used to clean the microwave glass and keypad. Be sure to remove the microwave from its enclave and clean under and around it.

Toaster: Most toasters have a slide-out platform under the toasting chambers. Remove that and clean the crumbs. Clean the surfaces of the toaster with glass cleaner.

Refrigerator/Freezer: Defrost the freezer by unplugging the unit. When it has defrosted, sponges dipped in a baking soda solution are great cleaners for the interior. A little vanilla extract can be added to the mixture to give the entire refrigerator a nice smell. Don't forget to clean the drip pan as well as the rest of the interior. When the unit is clean, leave an open box of baking soda to control food odors. One box will last approximately two months. Clean the outer doors with a cloth dipped in mild detergent, or if they're stainless steel, use a commercial stainless steel spray. And, don't forget to clean the rubber gasket seals around the doors with warm, soapy water. At least twice a year, use a vacuum cleaner attachment with a long-handled brush to clean the condenser coils in the bottom grill or kick plate, but be sure to unplug the appliance when doing this. This will increase the efficiency of the refrigerator by 3 to 5 percent, and that can result in savings of $100 or more in electricity costs each year. Finally, clean out any old food at the same time as cleaning the rest of the unit.

Sink: The sink will likely become dirty from this cleaning process as well as normal use. Wipe it out with hot, soapy water. Be sure to pay particular attention to the crevices in the backsplash and around the faucet. Use a disinfectant spray to remove stubborn stains.

Dishwasher: Use a baking soda and vinegar mixture to clean the dishwasher. This will remove the soap residue build-up that accumulates over time. Use a cup of vinegar mixed with one-half cup of baking soda and run the dishwasher empty.

Deep Cleaning the Bathroom

The bathroom is another challenging area to clean, but it is a particularly important area to maintain in pristine condition. To clean it, focus on the following areas:

Grout: There are a number of grout cleaners that are available for cleaning the bathroom grout, but it's also possible to make a solution using one part bleach to 10 parts water. Fill a spray bottle with that mixture and spray it on the shower floor and tiled walls. Pay particular attention to any visible mold. Let the solution sit for at least 5 minutes before gently scrubbing the mixture off with a scrubbing sponge or an old toothbrush.

Shower Curtain: This is another area where mildew accumulates. If the shower curtain is washing machine safe, it can be washed that way. If not, or to clean the plastic curtain behind a linen curtain, use a bathroom cleaner. If the plastic curtain becomes too full of mildew, they are inexpensive and can be easily replaced.

Toothbrush Holder: This is easy to overlook and often gets very dirty. Soak the toothbrush holder in hot, soapy water to soften the residue. Use soap, a pipe cleaner, a straw cleaner, or any other fine brush to scrub the inside of the holder. Once the grime has been removed, run it through the dishwasher or put it in boiling water for at least 30 seconds. It can also be left submerged in vinegar for 30 minutes or soaked in a 1:10 bleach solution for 30 minutes.

Toilet: Believe it or not, this can be cleaned in three minutes. For the first minute, open the lid and squirt in some commercial toilet bowl cleaner inside the bowl and around the rim. Close the lid and spray an all-purpose cleaner or disinfectant on the outside of the bowl. For the second minute, grab some paper towels and wipe down the back of the toilet, handle, top of the lid, the inside of the lid, and around the base. Microfiber towels are also great for this purpose, and they're good for picking up lint and germs, but they'll have to be washed afterward. In minute three, open the lid and use the toilet brush to scrub the inside of the toilet bowl--don't forget the inside of the rim. Flush the toilet and rinse the toilet brush. To get the hinges of the toilet seat clean, use an old toothbrush to scrub around them.

Deep Cleaning the Rest of the Home

With two of the worst areas for cleaning--the kitchen and the bathroom--scrubbed clean, it's time to deep clean the remainder of the home. This involves the following tasks:

- Cabinets/Drawers: Empty these out and use the vacuum to clean out any debris. Then, wipe the inside with a clean, wet rag or a cleaning spray. Wipe down the cabinet faces as well.
- Doors: Wipe down the doors, doorknobs, and door frames for fingerprints and smudges.
- Garbage cans: Wipeout and sanitize the garbage cans, recycling bins, and wastebaskets throughout the house.
- Blinds: For metal blinds, remove them and take them outside. Lay them on the patio and dip a brush in soapy water to scrub each side of the blinds. When clean, rinse them with a garden hose and dry them with a towel. Lay them in the sun to thoroughly dry them. Fabric blinds can be spot cleaned with an all-purpose cleaner using a rubber sponge. A vinegar solution also makes a good disinfectant cleaner.
- Faucets: Use vinegar to descale faucets and showerheads throughout the home, and be sure to clean out the aerators in the heads.

- Vent covers: Remove the HVAC vent covers throughout the home and wash them with warm, soapy water.

- Windows: Vacuum window sills and tracks, and remove cobwebs and bugs from the screens. Clean the windows with a window cleaner.

- Ceiling fans: Wipe down and clean the fan blades.

- Couch and Chairs: Remove the cushions, vacuum the creases, and move the couch to clean under and behind it.

- Carpet: Spot clean any stains on carpet and upholstery. There are a number of commercial upholstery cleaners available to use for this purpose.

- Dust and vacuum: Dust all surfaces including hard-to-reach ledges, windows, light fixtures, and the tops of cabinets and other fixtures. It's important to clean all of the places that are hard to get to during normal cleaning. As necessary, get out the stepladder to reach those high areas, but be careful not to fall.

Remember that if the cleaning process causes too much distress, there is no shame in hiring a professional cleaning service to do the deep cleaning. Many people who are not hoarders prefer to use professional cleaning services, and no one considers the fact that they do as a sign of failure. It's no different if a hoarder chooses to do the same. Just keep checking in with and processing any feelings that arise during the cleaning process. This is the final step in the decluttering process, and by this point, the goal of having a clean, organized home has been achieved. This is something to celebrate. Visit the vision board once again and post some pictures of the newly decluttered and clean home along with images of the happy faces of those who accomplished this goal. And, take the time to enjoy a reward, like a nice dinner or a fun activity.

Chapter Summary

This chapter presented information on the final deep cleaning once the decluttering process is complete. Specifically, the following topics were discussed:

- Suggestions for approaching a deep clean;
- The supplies needed;
- The deep cleaning process;
- Cleaning the kitchen;
- Cleaning the bathroom;
- Cleaning the remainder of the house.

The following chapter will present information on having a plan to stay on top of the clutter.

Once the home is decluttered and cleaned, it will be easier to maintain that cleanliness. To stay motivated to that end, it can help to keep those photos taken after the deep cleaning was finished handy as reminders of how nice the home looks when it's clean. That can also help to prevent a relapse into unhelpful, past hoarding behaviors. Now, the task becomes maintaining that level of cleanliness. As with the other stages in the decluttering process, it can be helpful to develop a system.

A system for cleaning consists of a routine that becomes habitual. Remember that creating a habit actually results in physical changes in the neural pathways of the brain. Once those pathways have been reinforced, the brain will actually create urges to engage in the habitual behavior. This is why it can be so difficult to overcome bad habits, but in this case, this mechanism is helpful for creating a good cleaning habit. To establish a habit, repetition is key, and one of the best ways to ensure repetitive cleaning behavior is to create a cleaning schedule.

Establish a Cleaning Schedule

People whose houses are always clean achieve those results by maintaining a systematic cleaning schedule. This can be divided into those tasks which are done daily, biweekly, and those which are done weekly. Then, there are also a few tasks that are done less frequently than that, but those go on the schedule too. The following is a sample schedule that can be adjusted for individual circumstances.

Daily focus and tasks: The daily focus is to keep dirt at bay. This type of cleaning will involve handling any messes that occur from normal living to prevent both dirt and clutter accumulation. This is something that helps keep everything tidy, but doesn't clean the more serious dirt. The tasks associated with daily cleaning are the following:

- Make the bed;
- Put any dirty clothes in the hamper;
- When there are enough clothes for a load of laundry, do it;
- Wipe the countertops after preparing meals;
- Wash dishes;

- Clean up clutter hot spots--these are the areas that seem to naturally accumulate clutter, like the entryway or kitchen countertops. By putting items away or discarding them daily from these areas, it will prevent significant clutter accumulation.
- Wipe out the kitchen and bathroom sinks.

Weekly focus and tasks: The focus here is a more thorough cleaning that focuses on those areas that don't require daily attention. Here are some tasks associated with weekly cleaning. These are spread throughout the week so that the task completed on any given day doesn't take much time:

- Sunday: Vacuum all carpets and rugs, and mop tile floors.
- Monday: Vacuum furniture.
- Tuesday: Wash bedsheets.
- Wednesday: Clean windows.
- Thursday: Clean bathroom.
- Friday: Clean stove.
- Saturday: Dust and wipe down surfaces to remove smudges.

Seasonal focus and tasks: The focus here is on deep cleaning. It doesn't have to be done very frequently, but when it is time, the focus is to remove grime from all areas that don't get much attention throughout the year. The entire house should be deep cleaned at least once a year, but it's also possible to divide that job into seasonal cleaning tasks. Here is an example.

- **Winter**: In December, clean out and wipe down all cabinets. When cleaning the medicine cabinet, dispose of unused or expired medications. In January, clean behind the refrigerator, washer, dryer, and all large furniture. In February, steam clean the carpets.

- **Spring**: In March, empty the closets and donate any unwanted or unused items. Re-organize the closet to prioritize clothes for the spring and summer seasons. In April, clean the window exteriors and screens. In May, wash blankets, comforter, duvets, and the remainder of any large bedding.

- **Summer**: In June, clean and organize the garage and/or basement. In July, empty, clean, and organize dresser drawers. Donate unwanted or unused items. In August, clean walls and retouch paint as necessary.

- **Fall**: In September, reorganize the closets and dressers for the upcoming colder seasons. In October, deep clean the refrigerator and freezer as

well as the stove and oven. In November,
consolidate and organize personal files.

By breaking up these deep cleaning tasks into monthly chores, it will make it much easier to follow through on the cleaning. Doing one task each month won't be as overwhelming as thinking about deep cleaning the entire house. There is room for flexibility, and of course, the schedule should be adjusted for individual circumstances, but once an appropriate schedule is in place, follow through on completing the tasks each month. Doing so will ensure the house stays clean and organized.

Here are a couple of other suggestions to maintain a clean, organized home.

Cleanliness Starts at the Door

Begin the process of keeping a clean, organized house at the front door. Leave shoes stored by the door and keep a pair of slippers to change into for wearing around the house. A mudroom entryway is a great help in keeping the house clean. That's where dirty shoes and outdoor clothing can be kept. That reduces the need to store those items in the main part of the house, and it prevents dirt from being tracked into the home interior.

A Place for Everything and Everything In Its Place

To keep an organized home, it's important to have a place to store everything down to the most minute detail. This includes things like keys, incoming mail (which should be sorted and disposed of as quickly as possible), and things like briefcases or other work-related items. Before bringing something new into the home, it is important to first ensure it has a proper place to be stored. If it doesn't, consider carefully whether it should be brought into the home.

One In, One Out Rule

This rule is just as it sounds--every time something is brought into the home, something else must be taken out. That helps to prevent duplicates and reduces the chance of building up significant amounts of clutter.

Stick to the Plan

Stick to the new organization system. Anything brought into the home should have a place to be stored, and it should fit in the individual system. If something is left on a free surface, it is important to stop and determine where it should go, and if, for that matter, it is something necessary to have. Complete daily and weekly tasks as scheduled.

Clean Frequently

It is important to keep the house clean to stay motivated to avoid clutter. This means cleaning frequently. In fact, for those areas that are used often, like the kitchen, it's important to clean them after every use. This is true for everyone, but it is particularly important for hoarders or someone living with a hoarder to be extra vigilant about this.

Miscellaneous Baskets

Create some miscellaneous baskets to collect objects throughout the day. Then, at the end of the day, return the items in those baskets to their permanent location. When relaxing, it's understandable not to want to put things away immediately, and that's where miscellaneous baskets can come in handy. Put items in the basket, and then before going to bed, take those items and return them to the proper storage area.

Filing Cabinet

A filing cabinet is a great item to have in the house in order to organize documents. This is where important documents can be easily organized and stored. When organizing the filing cabinets, label drawers in accordance with the types of documents that will be stored in each. For example, one drawer might be dedicated to financial documents while another is dedicated to titles and deeds. Still another might be dedicated to insurance documents. This will make it very easy to find these when necessary. A filing cabinet is not, however, a place to store junk mail. Be sure to get rid of that as soon as it comes in.

Impose Rules

Rules can ensure that the system will be followed. For example, one rule might be that there is no TV until the kitchen has been cleaned. Rules will help ensure that the home stays organized and there is little opportunity for clutter build up. By using rules to stay on top of the clutter, it won't get to a level that will be overwhelming.

Do It Now

Rather than putting a task off until a later time, it's a good practice to do it now. When it is evident that the task needs doing, completing it at that time will prevent a build of chores that need to be done. This doesn't work for every task, particularly those that need some planning or supplies, but for many things, like putting away that clutter, doing the task immediately can easily be done and that will help to prevent clutter build up.

Involve Family Members

Involving family members in the cleaning process can help make it go faster and in a much more enjoyable manner. One person should not be responsible for cleaning the entire house unless that person lives alone. If other people are living in the home, they should also have cleaning responsibilities. That helps keep everything clean and well-organized. Every family member should also be aware of the system and follow its guidelines.

Make Cleaning Fun

Cleaning and decluttering does not have to be a serious event. It can be fun. Turn on some mood music, light some candles, and dance around the room singing while cleaning. If kids are involved, turn the experience into a game with rewards for accomplishing the assigned tasks.

All of these tips can help turn cleaning chores into pleasant habits, and of course, they help prevent the build-up of clutter. With a plan to keep things clean and organized, the reward will be a beautiful, clean, and organized home that anyone would be proud to show off. That brings up one more suggestion--show off the clean, organized home. Make plans to host dinners or parties so that everyone can admire this clean, well-run home. That will provide both a reward for a job well-done as well as motivation to keep it clean.

Chapter Summary

This chapter presented information on having an organizational system for cleaning and decluttering regularly. Specifically, the following topics were covered:

- Establishing a cleaning schedule for daily, weekly, and monthly cleaning tasks:
- Organizational tips like the one in, one out rule and a place for everything and everything in its place;
- The importance of sticking to the plan and cleaning frequently;
- Imposing rules for cleaning and doing it now as well as making cleaning an enjoyable activity;
- Reward the accomplishment of a clean house by showing it off.

The next chapter will present information on continuing therapy for hoarding disorder and maintaining support networks.

Therapy is a key part of the treatment for hoarding disorder. Even after the decluttering process has been successful, it is vital to continue with supportive therapy. While it is easy for hoarders to think they've conquered the problem, therapy can help prevent relapses, which are common. Part of the problem common to a hoarder is something called cognitive disorganization.

Cognitive Disorganization

Research (Weir, 2020) indicates that there is a parallel between the hoarder's disorganized home and a disorganization in cognitive functioning. People who suffer from hoarding disorder demonstrate deficits in sustained attention, working memory, organization, and problem-solving. Additionally, they exhibit lower visuospatial ability. An individual's visuospatial ability is their capacity to identify visual and spatial relationships between objects. This means that hoarders have difficulty perceiving or mentally representing where objects are located in space, and they are unable to manipulate that knowledge in their spatial working memory. This negatively affects their ability to utilize that information to plan a sequence of movements.

These deficits in cognitive functioning are something reported by people with hoarding disorder frequently. They categorize it as difficulties with memory and being easily distracted. And, the degree of their own subjective impairment is correlated with their saving and acquiring behaviors (Weir, 2020). These cognitive problems appear to undermine the healthy reinforcement patterns that allow most people to let go of their possessions. For example, someone who doesn't cook much would have no problem giving up an unused griddle in their cupboard, but for someone with hoarding disorder, the griddle has a special meaning. The reinforcement pattern for the hoarder means that rather than associating the object with its usefulness, they attach special meaning to it, which makes it more difficult to discard. Attaching special meaning to objects isn't something that's unique to the hoarder, but hoarders are much more likely to apply sentimental meanings to almost every item then own. They are also much more likely to attach multiple meanings to each object. That further affects their ability to manage all of the associations they have with their possessions.

This cognitive disorganization displayed in people who suffer from hoarding disorder is visible with brain imaging technology. Scans using FMRI technology demonstrate that there is a lower connectivity evident in areas of a hoarder's brain associated with cognitive control. Moreover, there is greater connectivity in the default mode network, which is a brain network that becomes active as an individual's thoughts are focused inward as opposed to on the outside world. In comparisons of people with hoarding disorder, people with OCD, and healthy individuals in the process of making decisions about discarding their possessions, hoarders showed hyperactivity in the brain areas that compose what's called the salience network. This is the area of the brain that selects what stimuli are deserving of a person's attention. The same area of a hoarder's brain showed less activity than the other groups when considering other people's possessions. This indicates an overstimulation when it comes to considering discarding their own posses-sions, and it also suggests that those with hoarding disorder have difficulty making fine-grained decisions with regard to what is important. That's because their brain is always screaming that everything's important. Of course it would be difficult to discard any possession when this area of the brain is hyperactively insisting that everything is vital (Weir, 2020).

Treatment Options

This research serves to highlight the critical nature of continuous therapy to treat hoarding disorder. It will help the individual identify and address underlying psychological issues that tend to recur. With cognitive behavioral therapy, it is possible to identify and change the behavioral patterns that can lead to relapses, but that type of therapy takes time in order to treat the underlying causes of the behavior.

Cognitive Behavioral Therapy

CBT is by far the most successful method of treatment for hoarding disorder. There are a number of different applications of cognitive-behavioral therapy that can be useful in this regard. Some novel types of treatment include combining group cognitive behavioral therapy with online clinician support between therapy sessions. This method has shown promising results with higher group attendance and treatment gains that were maintained at the three-month follow-up assessment (Ivanov et al., 2018). Likewise, a blended therapy technique that involved twelve weeks of group therapy followed by eight weeks of online therapy showed promise in enhancing treatment effectiveness (Fitzpatrick et al., 2018). Other applications are specific to particular groups of hoarders. For example, a manualized CBT approach was used in a sample of geriatric patients with compulsive hoarding disorder. Though the results were limited in their efficacy, it highlights the need for innovative and population-specific treatments to this serious problem. The research indicates that problems with cognitive functioning are the underlying cause of hoarding disorder, and the higher frequency of cognitive impairment in this geriatric sample might explain the problems with this technique (Ayers et al., 2011).

The research into CBT for hoarding disorder indicates a significant decrease in symptoms with the best results obtained for discarding behaviors. But, despite positive results during the treatment process, most participants in the various studies on CBT treatments still showed significant hoarding behaviors after the treatment ended. This argues strongly for an ongoing treatment plan. While CBT is effective for reducing symptoms, it is not as effective as it is for other disorders like depression and anxiety. That indicates that CBT may not be the best option for every population. Younger people, for example, appear to benefit more from this treatment method than older people. That's a significant finding given that hoarding tends to get worse with age. For older adults, treatments modeled on interventions for individuals with traumatic brain injury may present a better option. In one study, participants showed a 40 percent reduction in symptoms with this kind of cognitive rehabilitation, and moreover, the improvements were maintained in a follow-up some six months after treatment (Weir, 2020). While still far from a cure, those results are encouraging, and also speak to the need for ongoing therapy.

Motivational Interviewing (MI)

Another type of treatment technique that is often used in conjunction with CBT is motivational interviewing. This technique attempts to increase the motivation of an individual to make positive changes in their behavior. It does that by helping individuals connect values and goals with behaviors. The technique also makes use of brainstorming different ways to change those behaviors which are not in line with the individual's goals and values. MI has proved to be a successful adjunct therapy for treating individuals with obsessive-compulsive disorder (OCD). It is specifically helpful in getting patients to adhere to a treatment protocol.

MI first seeks to develop a positive relationship between the therapist and the patient in order to reduce patient defensiveness and increase motivation for change. It is a person-centered method that seeks to help patients explore the reasons behind their reticence or ambivalence to treatment. For people who suffer from hoarding disorder, limited insight is a common characteristic, and many hoarders, therefore, demonstrate a level of ambivalence about their behavior. They may recognize that their behavior is creating problems, but they simply cannot bear to part with their possessions. Thus, their overall goals are at odds with their thinking. MI has proven to be particularly helpful in assisting patients with maintaining their motivation as they are participating in non-acquiring and discarding exercises.

MI has two primary goals, the first of which is to increase the importance of changing the behavior. This refers to addressing the discrepancy between the individual's current living environment and how they would like to live. They have to experience that discrepancy in order to be motivated to change. MI creates the discrepancy for them to experience by exploring their life goals and values while at the same time realistically examining their actual experience in their cluttered home. Often they have pushed aside their basic values as the clutter overtook their life. Thus, MI discussions about what they actually value the most in life help set the stage for determining the value of their possession within the context of how they would really like to live their life.

The second goal of MI is to increase the individual's confidence that they can change. This goal requires some careful, dedicated work in evaluating the value of those possessions as well as in experimenting with different ways to use, care for, and discard objects. By helping patients discuss and make plans for change, MI can help them make significant progress with CBT in reducing their hoarding symptoms.

Skills Training

Skills training is another essential adjunctive therapy for hoarding disorder. It seeks to help hoarders learn how to organize their belongings within their home, how to use problem-solving techniques to deal with common problems that arise as they go through the declutter process, and how to make decisions about what items are necessary to keep and what items can be discarded. The cognitive disorganization common to hoarders is what causes problems with decision-making skills. Therefore, giving hoarders a specific skill set for making decisions related to their possessions is a valuable adjunct to cognitive behavioral therapy.

Medication

Certain medications have a treatment value for those who suffer from hoarding disorder. These medications typically seek to change the brain chemistry and assist in the treatment for hoarding by reducing the anxiety and depression frequently experienced in various stages of therapy.

Outlook for Hoarding Disorder Treatment

The most successful treatment options for hoarding disorder are those that result from early recognition and diagnosis of the problem. That increases the likelihood that someone affected by this disorder can successfully reduce the severity of their symptoms. If left untreated, hoarding disorder is quite likely to become chronic and to get worse over time. For that reason, people exhibiting signs of hoarding disorder should speak with their doctor or mental health professional as soon as possible. For those who know someone that they believe is affected by this disorder, they should consider contacting a mental health professional to find out how they can help that person seek treatment. It's a complex problem that requires compassionate solutions.

Ongoing Therapy

Most of the research into the effectiveness of various therapeutic options indicates that the symptoms can be successfully reduced. But, the research also suggests the need for ongoing therapeutic support to maintain that reduction in hoarding behaviors. It's also important for individuals who suffer from this condition to maintain their support system that includes their family and friends. As part of the reward for decluttering, the individual can now host family and friends in their clean, well-organized homes. That's a powerful motivation for maintaining a clean, decluttered environment. Thus, family and friends can help by accepting those invitations and marveling at the progress made by the individual in dealing with this difficult condition. Social connections are powerful motivators for change.

Still, decluttering is only part of the solution. It's also vital that sufferers of hoarding disorder are able to address the underlying psychological elements that are ultimately the cause behind their behaviors. A strong support system that includes family, friends, and ongoing therapy is crucial for maintaining a decluttered lifestyle where the individual can feel safe and in control. It's important to not only declutter the home, but the mind as well. That's why treating the psychological and emotional aspects of hoarding is imperative to true, long-term success in treatment. A clean, organized environment is, for the hoarder, a journey, not a destination.

Chapter Summary

This chapter presented information on the importance of ongoing therapy for the successful, long-term treatment of hoarding disorder. Specifically, the following topics were discussed:

- Cognitive disorganization and its role in hoarding disorder;
- Treatment options;
- Cognitive-behavioral therapy, its effectiveness and variations;

- The role of motivational interviewing techniques in the treatment of hoarding disorder;
- Skills training and the treatment of hoarding disorder;
- The outlook for hoarders and the importance of ongoing therapy.

The next chapter will present concluding remarks.

FINAL WORDS

For the 2 to 5 percent of US adults who suffer from hoarding disorder, keeping a clean, organized environment is a struggle. Because of the accumulation of clutter that often reaches dangerous levels, these individuals also suffer from intense feelings of shame and isolation. They don't have what most people consider to be a normal life. They live amidst the uncontrolled clutter that is representative of the cognitive disorganization that is also common among those who suffer from hoarding disorder. The need to acquire new possessions is obsessive in these individuals, and the intense emotional attachment they form with those possessions makes it extremely difficult to engage in a declutter process.

There is, however, help for this disorder, and no one who suffers from this should feel alone. There are millions of people worldwide who display symptoms of hoarding. The treatment of this disorder requires a solid plan of attack for helping those individuals suffering as hoarders regain a level of control over their own behaviors. It involves setting manageable goals and taking the declutter process one step at a time. During the process, it is imperative to be mindful of the intense emotions that frequently arise and threaten to derail any progress.

This book has described 15 steps to take to reduce the clutter that so seriously affects those who suffer as hoarders. These steps are proven to be effective, and by breaking the process down into one step at a time, they are relatively easy to do. Among the tools described to help them are the following:

- Making a plan for decluttering;
- How to assess each item and determine whether it should be discarded, donated, stored, or displayed in the home;
- How to store memories without keeping objects;
- How to process the feelings of shame, guilt, and anxiety that inevitably arise during the declutter process.

By using the techniques described in the previous chapters, it is possible to clear out up to 80 percent of the items in the home, and this can be achieved with relatively little anxiety.

The aim of this book has been to present a compassionate and effective guide to help the most compulsive hoarder get their behaviors under control. And, more than simply the hoarding behaviors, it's imperative to address the underlying psychological issues that lead to hoarding in the first place. Toward that end, the previous chapters have described the variety of treatment options available to those who suffer as hoarders.

Among the most effective therapies available for hoarding disorder is cognitive-behavioral therapy. There are multiple goals of CBT, including understanding the root of hoarding behavior, utilizing techniques like motivational interviews to help them understand the discrepancy between their ideals and their real life experience. It aims to inspire change by allowing them to recognize that they are not living the life they want to live. And, once inspired, CBT can offer training in skills that are required for problem-solving and decision-making that many hoarders lack. With these skills, the hoarder will develop a greater ability to challenge their beliefs about their possessions, and that will allow them to assess their accuracy and make more appropriate decisions related to the object. Finally, for those hoarders who suffer severe anxiety during the declutter process, there are medications available to help alleviate those fears. Additionally, there are antidepressants that can help treat depression frequently experienced during the declutter process.

It is imperative to be patient in the decluttering process since the real work of the treatment is to address the underlying psychological issues. That's what will ultimately offer long-term relief. Following these guidelines will give hoarders and their loved ones the strategies they need to begin that journey of healing. This condition can be conquered, but it does take time, patience, and ongoing therapy to make progress. There are many people who have successfully made that journey using the strategies described in this book. It is possible to reclaim your life or help a loved one conquer this debilitating problem. The key is to stay positive, work the plan, don't be discouraged by setbacks, and keep moving forward. Anyone can benefit from these techniques. Really, it's about re-organizing your thoughts as much as your environment. There's no time like the present to get started on this difficult but rewarding journey. These techniques will help you regain the control you once had over your life and your environment. Get started implementing them today and get ready to say goodbye to the shame, the guilt, and the isolation this condition has caused. Say hello to your friends, your family, and your new organized, clean life.

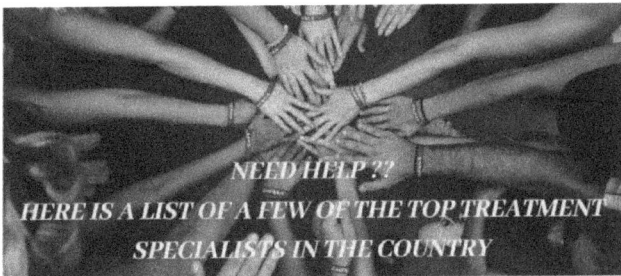
NEED HELP ??
HERE IS A LIST OF A FEW OF THE TOP TREATMENT
SPECIALISTS IN THE COUNTRY

THE LIST INCLUDES:

- *Nationally renowned treatment providers*
- *One-click linked portal access*
- *Locations and contact information*
- *Things to remember when seeking or providing help*

It's one thing to need help, and another to know where to go......

To receive your Renowned Treatment List, visit the link:

Renowned Treatment List

REFERENCES

ADAA. (n.d.). Hoarding: The Basics | Anxiety and Depression Association of America, ADAA. Retrieved April 8, 2020, from https://adaa.org/understanding-anxiety/obsessive-compulsive-disorder-ocd/hoarding-basics

AFIC Admin. (2018, December 30). What's The Difference Between Hoarding and Collecting? Retrieved April 17, 2020, from https://www.aifc.com.au/whats-the-difference-between-collecting-and-hoarding/

American Psychiatric Association. (n.d.). What Is Hoarding Disorder? Retrieved April 2, 2020, from https://www.psychiatry.org/patients-families/hoarding-disorder/what-is-hoarding-disorder

Anxiety Canada. (n.d.). Hoarding Disorder | Here to Help. Retrieved April 13, 2020, from https://www.heretohelp.bc.

ca/factsheet/hoarding-disorder

Anxiety Canada. (2019a, April 17). Challenge Negative Thinking. Retrieved April 13, 2020, from https://www. anxietycanada.com/articles/challenge-negative-thinking/

Anxiety Canada. (2019b, August 26). Helpful Thinking. Retrieved April 13, 2020, from https://www.anxietycanada. com/articles/helpful-thinking/

Ayers, C. R., Wetherell, J. L., Golshan, S., & Saxena, S. (2011). Cognitive-behavioral therapy for geriatric compulsive hoarding. *Behaviour Research and Therapy*, *49*(10), 689–694. https://doi.org/10.1016/j.brat.2011.07.002

Birchall, E., & Cronkwright, S. (2019, October 14). The Top 3 Hoarding Life Cycle Patterns: Is it true that people who hoard can't discard? Retrieved April 17, 2020, from https:// www.psychologytoday.com/us/blog/conquer-the-clutter/ 201910/the-top-3-hoarding-life-cycle-patterns

Bowen, A. (2019, August 19). When things become too much: How to help a hoarder. Retrieved April 13, 2020, from https://www.chicagotribune.com/lifestyles/health/sc-how-to-help-a-hoarder-health-0222-20170217-story.html

Budget Dumpster. (2020, November 4). How to Declutter Your Home: A Ridiculously Thorough Guide | Budget Dumpster. Retrieved April 11, 2020, from https://www.

budgetdumpster.com/resources/how-to-declutter-your-home.php

Clear, J. (2018, June 2). How to Stop Procrastinating by Using the '2-Minute Rule' Retrieved April 11, 2020, from https://medium.com/the-mission/how-to-stop-procrastinating-by-using-the-2-minute-rule-310fa8495fb9

Clear, J. C. (2019, February 1). How the 2-minute rule can help you beat procrastination and start new habits. Retrieved April 11, 2020, from https://www.cnbc.com/2019/02/01/the-2-minute-rule-how-to-stop-procrastinating-and-start-new-habits.html

Cleveland Clinic. (n.d.). Hoarding Disorder Management and Treatment. Retrieved April 11, 2020, from https://my.clevelandclinic.org/health/diseases/17682-hoarding-disorder/management-and-treatment

Cuncic, A. (2018, November 16). Understanding Cognitive Restructuring Core Part of Cognitive Behavioral Therapy. Retrieved April 11, 2020, from https://www.verywellmind.com/what-is-cognitive-restructuring-3024490

Firestone, L. (2018, October 18). Thinking Positively: Why You Need to Wire Your Brain to Think Positive. Retrieved April 13, 2020, from https://www.psychalive.org/thinking-positively/

Fitzpatrick, M., Nedeljkovic, M., Abbott, J.-A., Kyrios, M., & Moulding, R. (2018). "Blended" therapy: The development and pilot evaluation of an internet-facilitated cognitive behavioral intervention to supplement face-to-face therapy for hoarding disorder. *Internet Interventions, 12*, 16–25. https://doi.org/10.1016/j.invent.2018.02.006

Fortin, C., & Quilici, K. (2018, April 3). 9 Ways to Create a Realistic Plan to Declutter Your Home—And Stick to It. Retrieved April 12, 2020, from https://www. workingmother.com/9-ways-to-create-realistic-plan-to-declutter-your-home-and-stick-to-it#page-2

Golden, D. (2019, November 19). How to Overcome Hoarding. Retrieved April 13, 2020, from https://www. therecoveryvillage.com/mental-health/hoarding/related/how-to-overcome-hoarding/#gref

Grisham, J., & Baldwin, P. (2015). Neuropsychological and neurophysiological insights into hoarding disorder. *Neuropsychiatric Disease and Treatment*, 951. https://doi. org/10.2147/ndt.s62084

Grohol, J. M. (2009, October 26). Why "Sleeping on It" Helps. Retrieved April 13, 2020, from https://www. livescience.com/5820-sleeping-helps.html

Henry, A. (2019, July 12). Productivity 101: An Introduction to The Pomodoro Technique. Retrieved April 11, 2020, from https://lifehacker.com/productivity-101-a-primer-to-the-pomodoro-technique-1598992730

Holt, L. (2018, August 12). Downsizing and letting go of family memorabilia. Retrieved April 13, 2020, from https://www.lindaholtcreative.com/2018/08/downsizing-and-letting-go-of-family-memorabilia/

International OCD Foundation. (2020, February 19). Treatment of HD – Cognitive Behavioral Therapy (CBT). Retrieved April 17, 2020, from https://hoarding.iocdf.org/professionals/treatment-of-hd-cognitive-behavioral-therapy-cbt/

Ivanov, V. Z., Enander, J., Mataix-Cols, D., Serlachius, E., Månsson, K. N. T., Andersson, G., … Rück, C. (2018). Enhancing group cognitive-behavioral therapy for hoarding disorder with between-session Internet-based clinician support: A feasibility study. *Journal of Clinical Psychology, 74*(7), 1092–1105. https://doi.org/10.1002/jclp.22589

Kane, A. C. (2019, December 13). How to Make a Vision Board. Retrieved April 11, 2020, from https://christinekane.com/how-to-make-a-vision-board/

Larkin, E. (2019, May 15). How to Stop Hoarding Before It Starts. Retrieved April 13, 2020, from https://www.thespruce.com/6-quick-tips-to-control-clutter-and-stop-hoarding-2648657

Mayo Clinic. (2018a, February 3). Hoarding disorder - Diagnosis and treatment - Mayo Clinic. Retrieved April 11, 2020, from https://www.mayoclinic.org/diseases-conditions/hoarding-disorder/diagnosis-treatment/drc-20356062

Mayo Clinic. (2018b, February 3). Hoarding disorder - Symptoms and causes. Retrieved April 12, 2020, from https://www.mayoclinic.org/diseases-conditions/hoarding-disorder/symptoms-causes/syc-20356056

NHS website. (2018, October 3). Hoarding disorder. Retrieved April 8, 2020, from https://www.nhs.uk/conditions/hoarding-disorder/

Oppong, T. (2018, June 21). The Neuroscience of Change: How to Train Your Brain to Create Better Habits. Retrieved April 13, 2020, from https://medium.com/swlh/to-break-bad-habits-you-really-have-to-change-your-brain-the-neuroscience-of-change-da735de9afdf

Owen, K. (2020, January 20). Compulsive Hoarding Treatment. Retrieved April 11, 2020, from https://www.verywellmind.com/hoarding-treatment-2510619

Phillips, A. (2017, September 3). The Psychological Benefits of Writing Things Down. Retrieved April 11, 2020, from https://rubyconnection.com.au/insights/lifestyle/the-psychological-benefits-of-writing-things-down

Rider, E. (2015, January 12). The Reason Vision Boards Work and How to Make One. Retrieved April 11, 2020, from https://www.huffpost.com/entry/the-scientific-reason-why_b_6392274

Shaw, A. M., Timpano, K. R., Steketee, G., Tolin, D. F., & Frost, R. O. (2015). Hoarding and emotional reactivity: The link between negative emotional reactions and hoarding symptomatology. *Journal of Psychiatric Research*, *63*, 84–90. https://doi.org/10.1016/j.jpsychires.2015.02.009

Staff at Oprah.com. (2018, January 2). The Best Decluttering Advice We've Heard. Retrieved April 13, 2020, from https://www.huffpost.com/entry/the-best-decluttering-advice-weve-heard_n_5a0c8906e4b0b17ffce1ffb8

Step by Step Declutter. (n.d.). Setting Goals. Retrieved April 11, 2020, from https://www.step-by-step-declutter.com/setting-goals.html

The Oprah Winfrey Show: The Podcast. (2009, October 6). 12 Tips to Overcome Hoarding. Retrieved April 13, 2020, from https://www.oprah.com/home/how-to-overcome-hoarding/all

The Recovery Village. (2020, January 27). Hoarding Statistics. Retrieved April 2, 2020, from https://www.therecoveryvillage.com/mental-health/hoarding/related/hoarding-statistics/#gref

Tolin, D. F., Hallion, L. S., Wootton, B. M., Levy, H. C., Billingsley, A. L., Das, A., ... Stevens, M. C. (2018). Subjective cognitive function in hoarding disorder. *Psychiatry Research*, *265*, 215–220. https://doi.org/10.1016/j.psychres.2018.05.003

Vandenberg, S. (2019, July 1). How to clean a hoarder's house - Hoarding cleaning tips and steps. Retrieved April 12, 2020, from https://www.servicemastersanfrancisco.com/clean-hoarders-house/

Weir, K. (2020, April 1). Treating people with hoarding disorder. Retrieved April 17, 2020, from https://www.apa.org/monitor/2020/04/ce-corner-hoarding

Woods, R. (2020, November 4). How to Declutter Your Home: A Ridiculously Thorough Guide | Budget Dumpster. Retrieved April 11, 2020, from https://www.budgetdumpster.com/resources/how-to-declutter-your-home.php

Yap, K., Eppingstall, J., Brennan, C., Le, B., & Grisham, J. R. (2020). Emotional attachment to objects mediates the relationship between loneliness and hoarding symptoms. *Journal of Obsessive-Compulsive and Related Disorders*, *24*, 100487. https://doi.org/10.1016/j.jocrd.2019.100487

www.ingramcontent.com/pod-product-compliance
Lightning Source LLC
Chambersburg PA
CBHW031139020426
42333CB00013B/440